THE
HEADACHE
BOOK

THE HEADACHE BOOK

SEYMOUR SOLOMON, M.D.,
AND STEVEN FRACCARO

Consumer Reports Books
A Division of Consumers Union
Mount Vernon, New York

Library of Congress Cataloging-in-Publication Data
Solomon, Seymour.
The headache book / Seymour Solomon and Steven Fraccaro.
p.   cm.
Includes bibliographical references and index.
ISBN 0-89043-351-8
1. Headache—Popular works.   I. Fraccaro, Steven.   II. Title.
RB128.S64   1991
616.8′491—dc20   90-49894
CIP

Book design and composition by The Sarabande Press
First printing, April 1991
Manufactured in the United States of America

The diet chart on pages 89–93 is reprinted courtesy of Montefiore Medical
Center Headache Unit, Bronx, New York.

The Headache Book is a Consumer Reports Book published by Consumers Union, the nonprofit organization that publishes *Consumer Reports*, the monthly magazine of test reports, product Ratings, and buying guidance. Established in 1936, Consumers Union is chartered under the Not-for-Profit Corporation Law of the State of New York.

The purposes of Consumers Union, as stated in its charter, are to provide consumers with information and counsel on consumer goods and services, to give information on all matters relating to the expenditure of the family income, and to initiate and to cooperate with individual and group efforts seeking to create and maintain decent living standards.

Consumers Union derives its income solely from the sale of *Consumer Reports* and other publications. In addition, expenses of occasional public service efforts may be met, in part, by nonrestrictive, noncommercial contributions, grants, and fees. Consumers Union accepts no advertising or product samples and is not beholden in any way to any commercial interest. Its Ratings and reports are solely for the use of the readers of its publications. Neither the Ratings, nor the reports, nor any Consumers Union publications, including this book, may be used in advertising or for any commercial purpose. Consumers Union will take all steps open to it to prevent such uses of its materials, its name, or the name of *Consumer Reports*.

To my wife, Ethel
—S.S.

To the memory of my father, Albert Fraccaro
—S.F.

CONTENTS

ACKNOWLEDGMENTS

The authors wish to thank Richard B. Lipton, M.D., for his major contributions to chapter 2, "Tension Headaches," and for his valuable advice throughout the writing of this book.

THE
HEADACHE
BOOK

INTRODUCTION

I f you've picked up this book you probably suffer from headaches or know someone who does. The headaches may be a
new and disturbing intrusion in your life or, more likely, you may
have endured them for years. Perhaps you're temporarily disabled
by the pain, by its intensity or duration, or by the sheer frequency
of its occurrence.

Many of us perceive chronic pain as a matter over which we
have little or no control, and thus as a threat to our emotional and
mental stability. Indeed, if you experience headaches that are
frequent and severe, you may find it difficult to cope with daily
life and its challenges. As a further complication, people who
suffer from headaches are often regarded by others as neurotic
complainers or malingerers, and they may even begin to view
themselves in that light. This attitude is not only unjustified, it
can also be dangerous. Persistent or recurrent head pain may be a
signal of a serious illness, and if you suffer from chronic headaches you should seek reliable medical help without fail.

While headaches are among the most common of medical
complaints—studies estimate that only 10 percent or less of the
general population has *never* experienced a headache—their consequences can be severe. More than 40 million people in the

United States suffer from recurring headaches that interfere with their daily activities to some degree. We Americans lose more than 150 million work days per year because of headaches, at a cost to the economy of billions of dollars. Closer to home, the emotional stress imposed on headache sufferers, as well as on their families and friends, is immeasurable.

If it's any comfort, people who suffer from headaches are in good company. The list of historical figures who experienced severe and debilitating headaches reads like a *Who's Who* of Western civilization. It includes Julius Caesar, Saint Hildegard, Queen Mary I, Cervantes, John Calvin, Alexander Pope, Madame de Pompadour, Thomas Jefferson, George Eliot, Heinrich Heine, Edgar Allan Poe, Charles Darwin, Ulysses S. Grant, Leo Tolstoy, Sigmund Freud, George Bernard Shaw, Virginia Woolf, and countless others.

HEADACHE THROUGH HISTORY

Headaches have always been part of the human condition. One of the first written references to head pain is from a Babylonian poem of 3000–2000 B.C.:

> Headache roameth over the desert, blowing like the
> wind,
> Flashing like lightning, it is loosed above and below . . .

Egyptian papyrus manuscripts dating from 1550 B.C., but possibly based on even earlier sources, describe familiar headache symptoms, as well as record various exotic attempts at treating them. Ancient Greek and Roman writers make frequent references to head pain. Hippocrates, in the fourth century B.C., accurately described the visual hallucinations that may precede a migraine attack, as well as headaches brought on by sexual intercourse and other forms of physical exertion. Paul of Aegina, another ancient Greek physician and writer, described a form of headache attributable to "intemperance only."

The ancient belief that headaches were caused by demons or other supernatural sources accounts for many of the seemingly bizarre attempts that have been made to treat them through the ages. Certain of these "remedies" were far worse for the patient than the headache itself. Some anthropologists believe, for example, that prehistoric skulls showing evidence of drilled holes or trepanning belong to the unfortunate victims of attempted cures for head pain.

The Greek physician Aretaeus wrote an unmistakable description of migraine in the second century A.D., but little more was noted on the subject until Thomas Willis, a seventeenth-century British physician, commented on its prevalence. He observed that the headache was "a disease which falls upon . . . sober and intemperate, the empty and the full-bellied, the fat and the lean, the young and the old, yea, upon men and women of every age, state or condition." He described headaches brought on by wine, food, oversleeping, sitting in the sun, sexual activity, and "passion." What is most interesting for us is his view that head pain did not occur in the brain, but was caused by distended blood vessels that applied pressure on "the nervous fibers."

Modern medicine began to make progress in the understanding of headaches during the late nineteenth and early twentieth centuries, when much of the theoretical groundwork was laid for our current knowledge. The first systematic studies of the physical changes that take place during a headache were conducted in the 1930s and 1940s by Drs. Bronson S. Ray and Harold G. Wolff of New York Hospital. They performed a series of experiments with patients who were undergoing head surgery. Under a local anesthetic, the patients were able to report when and where they felt pain, allowing the researchers to determine which areas in the head were sensitive to stimulation and which were not. Drs. Ray and Wolff were able to demonstrate that the brain itself is not sensitive to pain, but that the tissues between the skull and brain, in particular the large blood vessels on the brain's surface, are distinctly sensitive to a wide variety of stimuli. Thus, the theory expounded by Thomas Willis some three centuries earlier—that an increase in the size of the blood vessels in the head might exert pressure on nerve cells and cause pain—was supported for the first time.

Since then, we have seen enormous advances in the study of headaches. During the 1950s, scientific attention was directed toward the biochemicals involved in the mechanism of headaches. In the 1960s and 1970s, cerebral-blood-flow studies made further important contributions to the understanding of this mechanism. With the increasingly sophisticated technology available during the 1980s, the biochemical, vascular, and neurological concepts of headaches were gradually integrated. It is this body of continuing research that forms the basis for this book.

HEADACHE TYPES

If you suffer from headaches or know people who do, you know that headaches come in a great variety. You may experience headaches several times a year, monthly, once or more a week, or even daily. A single headache may last for a few minutes or for many days. The pain itself may vary from a mild aching to a moderate throbbing to an excruciating sensation that is almost unbearable. It may be intermittent or constant. The pain may be located in the forehead or temple, near the eyes or the back of the head, or on one side of the head or on both sides. Certain types of headaches may be accompanied by other symptoms, such as nausea, vomiting, and troubling disturbances of mood and vision.

In order to understand and coordinate the wide variety of headache characteristics, physicians have developed a number of ways to classify head pain. The most important distinction is made between those headaches that are due to an underlying disease or injury—*organic headaches*—and those that are not. Organic headaches usually account for fewer than 10 percent of the headaches reported to physicians. They may be caused by conditions ranging from a simple bump on the head or a fever to a serious disease such as a brain tumor.

Nonorganic headaches account for more than 90 percent of headaches. The term *nonorganic* does not mean imaginary; it refers to those headaches that constitute a series of distinct conditions caused by changes in the physiology or functioning of certain areas of the head—particularly the blood vessels and muscles. This kind of pain is the body's response to a stimulus that alters function rather than an attack to the head's structure, as caused by an organic disease. Exactly why some of us react to a certain stimulus—emotional stress, for instance—by getting a headache, while others do not, is still a mystery.

The most common nonorganic headaches are *migraine* and *tension headaches*. *Cluster headache*, another major type of nonorganic headache, occurs less often.

USING THIS BOOK

In 1988 the International Headache Society published an up-to-date classification of all types of headaches, and established criteria for making diagnoses. Much of that data has been adapted for this book.

The chapters that follow describe migraine, tension headache, and cluster headache in depth, with a full examination of their characteristics, causes, and treatments, including current drug and nondrug therapies. You'll learn about the everyday factors that can trigger headaches and about those headaches that are the result of other medical conditions. Controversial issues relating to headaches are explored, as are the special cases of headaches in children and the elderly. The final chapter explains when and how you should seek professional medical advice, and what you can expect when you do.

You will probably recognize your own type of headache in these pages, and perhaps you will decide that you have learned here how to treat it yourself. *Do not rely on your own self-diagnosis.* In some cases, delay in getting medical help can be crucial. Your doctor is in the best position to diagnose your headache and to recommend treatment. The purpose of this book is to help you become an informed medical consumer, which means being able to communicate clearly with your physician and share in the responsibility for your treatment. In this way, you'll have the best ammunition to alleviate, if not totally eliminate, the pain and anxiety of a possibly debilitating and emotionally draining condition.

1

Migraine Headaches

The Greek physician Aretaeus, writing in the second century A.D., observed that what we call migraine today was characterized by pain located on the left or right side of the head, and was often accompanied by "unseemly and dreadful symptoms" such as nausea, vomiting, malaise to the point of collapse, anxiety, and an instinctive flight from light to darkness.

Not all migraine sufferers experience the same symptoms, but physicians over the centuries, starting with Aretaeus, have noted the one-sided nature of migraine headaches as a frequent and distinguishing characteristic. The Greek word for the disorder, *hemicrania* ("half head"), thus became *hemicranium* in Latin, shortened to *megrim* in Old English, and, eventually, *migraine* in French and modern English.

Migraine isn't simply a painful headache, but an entire syndrome, involving a one-sided, throbbing head pain and a range of other symptoms that almost always include nausea and a heightened sensitivity to light and sound. Other potential associated symptoms may include physical, visual, neurological, and psychological complaints. The headache itself can be moderate or severe, and usually lasts from three hours to as long as three days.

DIAGNOSIS

If you suffer from migraine, you may not have realized what was happening the first time you had an attack. Perhaps you experienced visual hallucinations before the headache began, or the accompanying nausea or vomiting may have been as disabling as the headache itself. And the aspirin or other over-the-counter medications you might have tried probably didn't help much.

Because migraine is defined as a *recurrent* disorder, a physician cannot make a diagnosis on the basis of a single initial attack. If, however, you've experienced several such attacks that seem to fit the migraine pattern, then your doctor has a reliable basis for interpreting your symptoms.

When a doctor suspects migraine, you will be asked if you remember any particular symptom that occurred a day or a few hours before your headache (a *prodrome*), or 20 to 30 minutes before the headache (an *aura*). Were you aware, too, of any factors that may have triggered the headache, such as emotional stress or eating a certain food? What did you do to help relieve the headache? (Most migraine sufferers instinctively lie down in a darkened room.) Has anyone else in your family ever experienced similar recurring headaches? Depending on your answers, the physician can decide whether your headaches fit the established criteria for migraine attacks, although not all of the following features need to be present for a diagnosis of migraine:

- one-sided pain
- a throbbing, pulsating quality of pain
- pain of moderate to severe intensity

- pain aggravated by activity
- presence of nausea, with or without vomiting
- increased sensitivity to light or sound

The facts that the headaches may be aggravated during the menstrual period and that other family members have similar headaches are considered major supporting evidence for the diagnosis of migraine.

VARIETIES OF MIGRAINE

The two basic types of migraine are *common migraine*, distinguished by the absence of an aura, or warning period, and *classic migraine*, which is preceded by an aura. The classic attack, because of the remarkable nature of the aura that precedes the headache, is the easiest to recognize, but it occurs in only 10 percent of patients with migraine. Most people with classic migraine have experienced common migraine as well. It is common migraine, without the aura, that occurs in the great majority of migraine patients.

COMMON MIGRAINE/
MIGRAINE WITHOUT AURA

Common migraine usually first appears in adolescence or young adulthood, although it may also begin in childhood or middle age. It is rare, however, for an initial migraine episode to appear after late middle age. After age 50 or so, migraine attacks usually occur less frequently and with less severity, and they often disappear altogether. The reason for this, at least in women, is thought to be related to the hormonal changes that are associated with menopause.

Migraine attacks are about four times more common among

women than among men. Changes in levels of estrogen and other female hormones may be a major factor. However, researchers have been unable to find consistent differences in the levels of the female hormones in women who suffer migraine compared to women who do not. We do know there is a genetic susceptibility to migraine, however. About 70 percent of people with migraine symptoms have other family members with this condition.

Early Warning Symptoms (The Prodrome)

While common migraine is distinguished from the classic variety of migraine by its lack of an aura (which occurs 20 to 30 minutes before the classic migraine headache), attacks of common migraine do not necessarily arrive completely without warning. Several hours or a day before the headache, the common or classic migraine sufferer may experience a variety of odd sensations, such as unusual fatigue, yawning, irritability, depression, or even a sense of euphoria. These early symptoms are known as the prodrome of migraine. Less frequent prodromes are a craving for certain foods, unusual thirst, or a general sense of weakness and lassitude.

Not everyone who suffers from migraine experiences all, or even any, of these prodromes, but the recurrence of one or more of them can help confirm the diagnosis. Sometimes the symptoms may be subtle and may be recognized only after a number of attacks have occurred. Many patients eventually come to anticipate their attacks by the onset of certain prodromal symptoms.

Pain: Location, Severity, and Quality

The pain of common migraine, as noted earlier, is typically located on one side of the head, most often around the temple. Sufferers usually describe it as "throbbing" or "pulsating," and of moderate to severe intensity. These characteristics vary, however. Some migraine sufferers may experience brief jolts of momentary pain, while others describe a steady ache. The pain may switch from one side to the other or may be felt on both sides. (Headaches on both sides of the head have been reported in up to one-third of migraine sufferers.) Some patients have headaches that start in the back of the neck and radiate to the forehead, or vice versa. Stiffness or tenderness of the neck may also be present. The variation in symptoms can be considerable.

Duration and Frequency

The duration of the common migraine may vary from several hours to three days or, in rare cases, longer. When a migraine lasts longer than 72 hours, the condition is referred to as *status migrainosus*, a condition that always warrants medical attention and may require hospitalization (see page 43).

The frequency of migraine attacks also varies enormously. Some people with common migraine suffer only a few episodes in their lifetimes. Others may endure several attacks a week. The average frequency is one to three attacks per month. Episodes may occur at any time of day or night; many migraine patients report awakening in the morning with a headache.

Associated Symptoms

Nausea and vomiting. If your headache is diagnosed as common migraine, it will be accompanied by other symptoms in addition to head pain. Nausea for example is experienced by almost all patients with common migraine. Vomiting, diarrhea, or abdominal cramps may also occur. At times, the nausea and vomiting may be more disturbing than the actual headache; sustained vomiting can cause fluid and mineral loss, resulting in weakness and exhaustion. Some patients report that their vomiting seems to stop the migraine attack, but it's not clear whether the vomiting is the cause or the result of an attack's conclusion. Occasionally, loss of appetite occurs rather than nausea. In rare cases patients become acutely hungry, sometimes craving specific foods.

Sensitivity to light and sound. Increased sensitivity to light (*photophobia*) and to sound (*phonophobia*) are common symptoms of migraine, and patients report that light and sound appear to increase the severity of their pain. This sensitivity explains why migraine sufferers instinctively seek out a darkened quiet room, and why they find even relatively innocuous sounds enormously irritating. This heightened awareness may also apply to odors — perfume or cooking odors, no matter how mild, can often aggravate the attack.

Other physical changes. During an attack of migraine, the eyes and face may appear swollen, but more often the face is pale, sometimes to the point of being white or "ghostly." Paradoxically, some patients may develop a ruddy complexion. The eyes may become reddened or tear. The scalp is often tender, and the veins or arteries in the area of the temple may visibly swell or pulsate. The hands and feet of migraine sufferers are usually cold and clammy, even between attacks. The neck may feel stiff or tender to the touch.

Increased frequency of urination or an urge to have a bowel movement sometimes occurs during an attack. The sufferer may alternately feel hot and cold, but an actual fever is rare. A vague blurring of vision, dizziness (imbalance or lightheadedness), or a feeling of faintness may be noted.

Psychological effects. Emotional disturbances are common during an attack. These can include difficulty in remembering or in concentrating, anxiety, general nervousness or irritability, depression, and fatigue.

Resolution

When the attack subsides, most people feel completely exhausted. Some patients report a feeling of relief or even elation afterward, while others are depressed. The feelings of exhaustion or euphoria after an episode of migraine are related to changes that take place in the brain, in particular, to the activity of nerve cells and certain chemicals, especially those that act as *neurotransmitters*, or chemical messengers between nerve cells. Precisely why some people feel exhausted or depressed at the conclusion of an attack while others feel relieved or euphoric is not known. In addition, any of the prodromal symptoms may also occur during the resolution phase of the migraine.

No one experiences *all* of the symptoms described. The following records a typical case of common migraine:

Jane M., a lively and good-humored high school student of 16, began to experience headaches when she was 13. A severe, throbbing pain would develop rapidly in her right temple, and within an hour or two, it would spread across her entire head. Usually it lasted all day, and sometimes for two or even three days. Once it subsided, she felt exhausted.

While Jane invariably felt extremely nauseated during these headaches, she did not vomit. She found light, noise, and even pleasant odors such as flowers uncharacteristically irritating. She also experienced lightheadedness, perspiring hands, abdominal cramps, and sometimes diarrhea during the attacks. Her headaches occurred approximately three times a month.

These headaches often announced their arrival by awaking Jane in the morning, and at least one of the three each month would occur during her menstrual period. Emotional stress also seemed to be a precipitating factor; almost every time she argued with her boyfriend, for example, she would develop the headache once she returned home and tried to relax. She also noticed that she seemed to have more headaches on weekends and during summer vacations than she did during school. Missing a meal could also trigger an attack, as could eating hot dogs. When tested, however, Jane demonstrated no particular food sensitivities.

When Jane was experiencing these attacks, she wanted to be left alone, in darkness and silence. She would go immediately to her room, draw down the shades, and refrain entirely from playing the music she otherwise always enjoyed when resting. She also requested that her family remain as quiet as possible. Jane's older sister, who was away at college, experienced similar headaches, as had some of her aunts and uncles on her mother's side of the family. (They consoled Jane by telling her that the headaches would subside when she reached middle age.) General and neurological examinations were normal. The diagnosis was migraine without aura (common migraine).

Jane's older relatives had accepted their migraines in stoical fashion, regarding them as exasperating but familiar interruptions in their lives. With the benefit of diverse therapies that weren't generally available when her relatives were her age, Jane and her doctor gradually were able to control her migraine attacks.

CLASSIC MIGRAINE/MIGRAINE WITH AURA

Classic migraine is distinguished from common migraine by the *aura* (visual or other neurological disturbances) that precedes the headache by some 20 or 30 minutes. (Sometimes symptoms of the aura persist into, or initially occur during, the headache phase.) The aura should not be confused with the prodrome, which comes hours or a full day before the headache and is not as dramatic. The headache of classic migraine is often of briefer duration and less severe than that of common migraine. Otherwise, attacks of classic migraine may include all the phases of common migraine: the prodrome, the headache and associated symptoms, and the resolution phase. As with common migraine, not all episodes of classic migraine are preceded by the prodrome. To be diagnosed as classic migraine, however, they must be preceded by an aura. Thus, a typical classic attack would follow this sequence:

- prodrome
- aura
- headache phase, with accompanying symptoms
- resolution

The Aura

The presence of an aura before the headache is so important that the diagnosis of classic migraine may be made even if the subsequent headache and accompanying symptoms do not follow the same pattern as those described under common migraine. (Rarely do symptoms of the aura occur during the headache, but almost always before the headache begins.) Although any neurological symptom may occur as an aura, visual symptoms are by far the most common.

The visual symptoms that most frequently constitute the aura of classic migraine have been responsible for numerous vivid and bizarre reports over the centuries. Saint Hildegard, a nun and visionary who lived in twelfth-century Germany, left written descriptions and drawings that are almost certainly records of her migraine auras. Other writers, often physicians, have left less poetic but more specific records. In 1892 Dr. William Gowers reported:

> One patient . . . with characteristic headaches preceded by hemianopia [loss of vision on one side] complained of bright stars before the eyes whenever she had looked at a brilliant light; and sometimes one of the stars, brighter than the rest, would start from the right lower corner of the field of vision, and pass across the field, generally quickly, in a second, sometimes more slowly, and when it reached the left side would break up and leave a blue area in which luminous points were moving.

Such extraordinary visual experiences are sometimes termed *pseudohallucinations*. (The person who experiences a true hallucination believes that what he or she sees is real. Most people who experience a migraine aura do not mistake what they see or feel for reality.) Nevertheless, considering the extreme nature of some of the visual and other symptoms associated with the aura, it's not surprising that an occasional person who experiences a first attack of classic migraine fears he or she is losing touch with reality.

The visual symptoms of the classic migraine aura are produced by a disturbance of the occipital lobe, the back part of the brain that interprets visual information. The fact that the visual effects of the aura have been reported even in migraine sufferers who are blind supports this concept.

The most common visual aura is called a *positive scotoma* and is experienced by the sufferer whether the eyes are open or closed. This scotoma consists of bright lights that often flash on and off. It typically appears as an arc of zigzag lines in a herringbone pattern, or what is known as *fortification spectra*, since the effect has been likened in appearance to the walls of a medieval fortress as seen from above. Within the arc may be a *negative scotoma*, or blind spot. The negative scotoma may take the form of blindness affecting the right or left half of the field of vision of both eyes. Other strange visual effects have also been recorded. For instance, objects may appear to change in size or shape or break into a mosaic pattern. An accurate as well as creative representation of some of these visual auras may be seen in the original drawings made by John Tenniel for Lewis Carroll's classics, *Alice in Wonderland* and *Through the Looking Glass*. Carroll, who experienced attacks of classic migraine, assisted the artist in his renderings.

Although visual symptoms are the most common, the aura may consist of any neurological symptom. Numbness, tingling, or other unusual sensations, as well as weakness and diverse disturbances of body function may occur. The numbness and tingling usually are confined to one side of the face and felt in the hand and arm on that side. Occasionally, weakness or temporary paralysis affects an entire half of the body. Difficulty in speaking, lack of coordination, confusion, and changes in mood also may occur.

The onset of an aura is gradual, in contrast to the symptoms of a stroke, which usually develop quickly. In rare cases, the aura may be maximal at the time of onset. The effect of the aura is often extremely disturbing. The migraine sufferer may feel powerless as the effects worsen: The flashing positive scotoma and the negative scotoma, or blind spot, slowly increase in size; other symptoms may occur, gradually spread, grow more prominent, and then disappear. The aura generally evolves over 20 to 30 minutes.

Associated Symptoms

The symptoms that accompany the headache phase of classic migraine may be the same as those seen in common migraine—nausea, vomiting, increased sensitivity to light and sound—but these symptoms are not as important in making the diagnosis as in cases of common migraine. Classic attacks tend to resolve more quickly than common attacks, and they rarely last more than 12 hours. Moreover, the resolution of the classic attack is often more abrupt.

A typical example of classic migraine is the case of Elaine A.:

The patient, a 31-year-old attorney in good health, has experienced severe headaches since she was 20. For a day or two before the headache occurs, she tends to yawn a great deal and to also crave sweets. She did not report these symptoms as the prodrome of the headache until she was specifically asked about them, whereupon she recognized them as regularly signaling the syndrome that would soon follow.

Twenty or 30 minutes before the onset of her head pain, she experiences an aura, which begins as a small arc of bright zigzag lines that appear to the left of whatever she is looking at. The arc grows larger and larger as the lines flash on and off. Within the arc, her vision is blotted out—she cannot read, for example, because the left half of the text is missing. These symptoms were initially very frightening to her until she became accustomed to their transient nature and to the fact that they heralded a headache.

She described the headache itself as a pulsating, throbbing pain of moderate to marked severity over both temples. The pain often spreads into the left eye and over the entire left half of the head. Along with the head pain, she experiences nausea and, when the headache is particularly severe, vomiting. Normal levels of light and sound are extremely unpleasant, and she feels anxious and irritable during the episode.

Many of her attacks seem to have no obvious cause but others are precipitated by eating chocolate. Missing a meal or oversleeping may also bring on an attack. During the headache, she feels best when lying down in a dark, quiet room, alone and undisturbed. She reported that her mother and her maternal aunt also suffered from recurring, one-sided, throbbing headaches but did not experience the aura.

Physical and neurological examinations were normal. A computerized tomogram (CAT scan) of the head was also normal. Even though the headaches affected both sides of the patient's head, the presence of the aura indicated a diagnosis of classic migraine.

Varieties of Classic Migraine

Scientists have distinguished certain subcategories of classic migraine according to the specific nature of the aura. These varieties of migraine are uncommon or rare. If paralysis or altered sensation occurs on one side, the term *hemiplegic migraine* is used. When symptoms implicate the areas in the back of or below the cerebral hemispheres of the brain (the brain stem or cerebellum), the condition is classified as *basilar migraine*. These symptoms include some of the following: incoordination, slurring of speech, vertigo, double vision, blindness of both eyes, decreased hearing, ringing in ears, depressed consciousness or confusion, weakness or numbness of right and left extremities. Hemiplegic migraine occurs in children. Basilar migraine develops mainly in children and adolescents.

Sometimes the aura occurs without the headache. This variety is termed a *migraine equivalent*, and while it may appear at any age, it is more common in middle-aged and older patients. People who have experienced classic migraines for many years may eventually have their full attacks replaced by a migraine equivalent after age 50 or so.

Retinal migraine is diagnosed when migraine is accompanied by blindness or blurring in one eye. *Ophthalmoplegic migraine* is a migraine headache associated with double vision that is attributed to the weakness of an eye muscle. Like hemiplegic and basilar migraine, it is most commonly observed in children and adolescents. Retinal migraine and ophthalmoplegic migraine sometimes do not precede the headache but may accompany or follow it and the eye symptoms may continue long after the headache has disappeared.

When the aura lasts into and beyond the headache phase, physicians use the term *complicated migraine*. This category has been further defined as *migraine with prolonged aura* (lasting up to seven days) and *migrainous infarction*. The latter refers to symptoms that last longer than one week or may be permanent; in such cases, the patient is considered to have suffered a stroke caused by migraine. This is a very rare condition.

MIGRAINE TRIGGERS

If you suspect migraine and consult a physician, the doctor will compile from your history a list of factors that seem to precipitate your migraine attacks. These are known as *migraine triggers* (see chapter 4).

Patients report a variety of conditions and events that seem to precipitate their migraine attacks. Bear in mind, however, that such an association does not necessarily imply a cause. Sometimes it is difficult to determine whether a particular factor (a specific food, for instance) triggers the attack or simply exacerbates the developing episode. Nevertheless, many common external and internal factors seem to trigger migraine and have been observed in a large number of patients, thus permitting certain generalizations.

The fact is that almost any change in the body or the external environment can trigger a migraine episode. Circumstances that most often precipitate migraine include emotional stress, menstruation and other hormonal changes, certain foods, alcohol, and alterations in sleeping or eating patterns. Someone who experiences recurring migraine attacks is not necessarily affected by any of these factors; an individual susceptibility must be present.

Although susceptibility is the most important factor, other considerations also play a role. In many cases a combination of factors occurring at the same time, or a greater than normal exposure to a single specific trigger, is necessary to provoke an attack. For example, eating a piece of chocolate in a peaceful setting may not set off an attack, but consuming an entire box of chocolates after a period of stress may do so.

Emotional Stress

There is no such thing as a life without stress. Nevertheless, it is also clear that prolonged emotional stress, whether self-induced or created by a particularly difficult environment, does play a role in disease.

As far as migraine is concerned, emotional stress can certainly provoke an attack. Many patients report that their attacks commence soon *after* the specific stress has abated rather than during the stressful episode. One possible explanation is that during stress all muscle tone, including that of blood vessels, is heightened. The relaxation in tone that follows stress allows blood vessels to dilate while the body as a whole attempts to relax.

Depression and anxiety may be associated with migraine, but they rarely trigger individual attacks. Overexcitement can be a precipitating element for many people, particularly children. Some authorities, in fact, have described migraine as a reaction of certain elements of the nervous system to overstimulation.

Menstruation and Hormonal Changes

As we have noted, some 75 percent of migraine sufferers are women. Since hormones play a major role in body function, it isn't surprising that they also have an effect on migraine. Paradoxically, both increases and decreases in estrogen levels in women have been thought to be associated with migraine attacks.

The relationship of menstruation to migraine is well established, if not fully understood. It's common for young women to report a first migraine attack around the time of their first menstrual period. In fact, the majority of women with migraine suffer attacks either immediately before, during, or immediately after their menstrual periods. Many also report that the migraine attacks they experience during menstruation are more severe than those that occur at other times, and a substantial number of women report migraines *only* during menstruation. The rapid lowering of estrogen levels that occurs during the menstrual period is thought to be a major factor in the increased frequency and severity of attacks. But medications used to counter these changes—such as the female hormone estradiol or the synthetic male hormone danazol—are not always helpful in preventing attacks.

Since menstruation has an effect on migraine, you would expect that other factors affecting estrogen levels also play a role. Paradoxically, migraine seems to be triggered by high estrogen blood levels as well as by their rapid drop. Oral contraceptives, which increase blood levels of estrogen, have been associated with migraine. In fact, many women stop taking birth control pills because of the headaches they experience while using them. Physicians usually advise women with migraine to discontinue oral contraceptives and employ an alternative form of birth control, but this recommendation is not absolute. It's definitely recommended, however, that you stop using the pill if your migraines grow more severe, more frequent, or can't be controlled with appropriate therapy. Neurological symptoms such as weakness or numbness in the limbs require the immediate discontinuation of oral contraceptives, as these symptoms may be the prelude to a stroke.

Women with migraine react variably to pregnancy and to the onset of menopause. During the first three months of pregnancy, the incidence of headaches may increase, but migraine attacks usually lessen or disappear during the second and third trimesters. Migraine also often tapers off around the time of menopause, an outcome that may be part of the general abatement of attacks that often takes place as the sufferer grows older. Women who take estrogen supplements after menopause sometimes report an increase in the frequency and/or severity of migraine attacks. If this should happen, and estrogen supplementation is necessary for medical reasons (such as the prevention of osteoporosis), the estrogen should be administered in low doses. Only a minority of women report an increase in their migraine attacks during menopause.

Diet

Diet has long been known to play a role in triggering migraine attacks. The mechanisms by which it does so are not clear, but it is generally agreed that certain foods do trigger attacks in some 8 to 10 percent of patients.

Indeed, many patients are convinced that their headaches are directly "caused" by eating certain foods. A host of foods and beverages have been associated with the onset of attacks, but not the same substances in all patients. As a rule, it is wise to avoid the foods and drinks that you associate with attacks. But what components of the foods might actually trigger the attack is still a matter for investigation.

Foods. Many foods containing the amino acid tyramine or other naturally occurring proteins have been associated with the onset of migraine attacks. Chief among the foods that include these substances are aged cheeses, liver, kidneys, and other organ meats, herring, yogurt and sour cream, beer and red wine, broad beans, chocolate, and nuts. Other amines implicated in migraine are phenylethylamine in chocolate and l'octopamine in citrus fruits.

Flavor enhancers and preservatives. Nitrites and monosodium glutamate (MSG) are other commonly consumed dietary substances. They are potential vasodilators and may trigger migraine by that action. Nitrites are substances that are used as color enhancers and preservatives in cured meats such as hot dogs, sausages, bacon, and ham. MSG is a flavor enhancer commonly used in Chinese cooking and in many prepared food products. MSG can cause a reaction that includes headache, sweating, and tingling of the upper body—the so-called Chinese restaurant syndrome. The symptoms have some resemblance to those accompanying migraine. The artificial sweetener aspartame (NutraSweet) has also been implicated as a migraine trigger.

Alcohol. The consumption of excessive amounts of alcohol can produce a headache in virtually anyone. Moreover, alcohol is a substance that has definitely been associated with triggering or exacerbating migraine. It acts to expand the blood vessels in the head and, when this occurs, may initiate a series of physiological changes that can lead to a migraine episode.

In someone who is susceptible, drinking even a small amount of alcohol may trigger a migraine attack. Red wine, in particular, is frequently reported as the offending agent, a double suspect as it contains tyramine as well as alcohol.

Caffeine. Caffeine is a substance that plays a dual role in headache. A strong cup of coffee may help to relieve a single attack, and caffeine is often added to pain relievers to enhance their action; it may help relieve migraine by its blood-vessel-constricting properties. On the other hand, through a rebound mechanism, the excessive use of caffeine can cause migraine to evolve into daily headaches (see chapter 2).

If you are accustomed to drinking many cups of coffee every day, and if you discontinue doing so, you may experience this rebound effect. The headache mechanism, suppressed by the caffeine, is released as the level of caffeine in the blood drops. This sequence of events has been suggested as one explanation for migraines experienced on weekends or vacations, when many people tend to drink less coffee than they do when at work.

Medications

A variety of medications have been implicated in triggering headaches in migraine sufferers, in particular, those drugs that act by dilating the blood vessels. Commonly included in this category are nitroglycerin, reserpine, hydralazine, and other drugs used in the treatment of heart disease and high blood pressure. These medications can also set off headaches through their actions on the nervous system. We have already noted that oral contraceptives and estrogen supplements can trigger migraine in some women.

Other medications used regularly to treat a variety of conditions can trigger headaches when *withdrawn*, or when their levels in the blood fluctuate. A rebound effect, for instance, may occur in people who take pain medication every day. Ergotamine tartrate, an important drug used to treat migraine, can cause headaches if it is used daily or almost daily in greater than prescribed doses (see chapter 4).

Miscellaneous Triggers

Changes in eating and sleeping patterns have also been targeted as migraine triggers. Fasting for 8 to 12 hours or longer has been found to provoke migraine: the longer someone refrains from eating, the more likely an attack. This result was once attributed to the reduced blood levels of sugar that come with fasting. But it has been established that, while fasting may lower the amount of sugar in the blood in patients who suffer from hypoglycemia, this condition is rare in nonhypoglycemic patients. We know that fasting or missing a meal causes other, not yet fully understood, biological changes that trigger the migraine. In any case, scheduling meals regularly may be helpful in preventing migraine attacks.

Many of the changes in the brain and body that take place during sleep might be responsible for a headache. These include alterations in the brain's blood flow and in the levels of certain chemicals necessary for the functioning of the brain and nervous system. Among the body chemicals most often implicated in migraine are epinephrine (adrenaline), norepinephrine (noradrenaline), and serotonin, all of which act as neurotransmitters—that is, chemical messengers between nerve cells.

It's possible that dreaming may set off a migraine. More commonly, disruptions in customary sleep patterns, including both too little or too much sleep, as well as changes in times of awakening and going to sleep, have also been implicated as triggers of migraine headaches. Eating regularly and going to sleep and awakening at the same time every day (including weekends) may help to control migraine episodes.

Weather is another factor that can trigger migraine. Hot, humid conditions (more often than cool, dry weather) are often reported to trigger migraines. Changes in atmospheric conditions may also set off an attack, but the actual mechanism is not known.

A number of other external physical factors are associated with setting the scene for a migraine attack. Sunlight or a light that glares or flickers can trigger attacks in some susceptible people. Strong odors or noise may generate or aggravate migraine. Traveling by airplane (the altitude) or by car (the motion of bumping up and down) are also common aggravating factors. Being struck on the head can provoke migraine episodes, particularly in children. The injury need not be severe; for example, a soccer ball hitting the head ("footballer's headache") may be sufficient to trigger migraine.

PERSONALITY AND MIGRAINE

Over the years, some physicians have attempted to define what is sometimes called a "migraine personality." They summarized certain character traits commonly seen in their migraine patients to produce a composite portrait of a compulsive perfectionist, a person who is both highly self-critical and particularly hard on others. But a substantial number of migraine patients do not conform to this stereotype; migraine sufferers range widely in character and behavior traits.

It should be noted that the so-called migraine personality bears a distinct resemblance to the "Type-A" personality that was so much in the news a few years ago and identified men at risk for heart disease. Similarly, the migraine profile is insufficiently specific—many people who do not fit the profile suffer from migraine; many others who may well fit such a profile have never experienced a migraine attack. Furthermore, because so many of us have a tendency to repress our emotions, it is exceedingly difficult for physicians to dig out and identify specific underlying emotional factors in migraine sufferers. For example, a patient who doesn't realize—or refuses to admit—that he or she is angry at a spouse or an employer may not be able to provide accurate answers to a physician's queries—assuming the physician takes the time to inquire patiently about such matters in the first place.

This reservation doesn't mean that the issue of emotional involvement should be totally ignored. Even if the exact mechanism isn't fully understood, stress clearly plays a role in migraine.

HEREDITY AND MIGRAINE

Based on statistical evidence, migraine is considered an inherited disorder. Only 16 percent of the general population report a close relative who suffered from migraine, compared with at least 60 percent of migraine patients who had relatives similarly affected. Among those who reported a family history of migraine, 53 percent had a mother with migraine, 17 percent a father, 17 percent a sister, and 12 percent a brother. Thus, migraine appears to be a genetically transmitted condition often inherited from the mother.

Because a specific gene for migraine has not yet been discovered, some researchers believe that the familial relationship might represent a learned response—to emotional stress, for example—rather than an inherited trait. The majority of physicians, however, believe that the genetic transmission of migraine, particularly from the maternal side, is well established.

MIGRAINE IN CHILDREN

Children may experience migraine in either its classic or common form. In contrast to the female predominance in adults, migraine that occurs before puberty is equally distributed between both sexes.

Unfortunately, particularly in the case of classic migraine, children are often ridiculed and disregarded when they describe the bizarre symptoms of an aura. Some patients who have suffered classic attacks since childhood report that they refrained from telling anyone about their episodes because they feared disbelief and derision from family and friends.

Children often experience symptoms that are precursors of, or associated with, future migraine attacks. Repeated bouts of periodic nausea and vomiting, without headache, sometimes develop into full-blown migraine episodes in later years. Similarly, periodic abdominal pain, without headache, may represent an early form of migraine in children, as may repeated cycles of vertigo. It's also interesting to note that adult migraine sufferers often report a history of car or motion sickness during childhood.

Because some of these childhood attacks follow emotional excitement or stress and seem to have no apparent physical cause, parents or physicians often wrongly consider them to be of psychological origin. It's important, therefore, that children who suffer recurrent bouts of such symptoms be evaluated with the diagnosis of migraine in mind (see chapter 8).

THE UNDERLYING CAUSES OF MIGRAINE

What changes in the body actually *cause* a migraine attack? What physiological events take place during a migraine episode? These questions are still being studied. While we have no complete answers, researchers have a fairly clear perspective about what mechanisms in the body contribute to the phenomena of migraine. (The relationship of migraine to tension headache is discussed in chapter 2.)

Vascular Factors

For many years, migraine was viewed as a predominantly vascular phenomenon. Investigators believed that it occurred when certain blood vessels in the brain first constricted, producing the aura of classic migraine, and then other blood vessels in the scalp dilated, producing the throbbing headache.

Although we know today that changes in the size of blood vessels do indeed take place during a migraine attack, researchers have recently focused more closely on events in the brain that *precede* these vascular changes. Nevertheless, a brief look at what happens to blood vessels during a migraine episode will be helpful in understanding the roles that both the nervous system and blood vessels play in producing the attack.

We have noted that it was Dr. Thomas Willis, a seventeenth-century British physician, who first proposed that migraine was caused by the swelling of blood vessels in the head. During the late nineteenth and early twentieth centuries, various researchers elaborated on this theory. Harold G. Wolff and his associates demonstrated that scalp vessels did indeed dilate during a migraine attack, thus supporting the vascular theory of migraine.

But in itself the dilation of the blood vessels of the head does not cause pain. Such changes are common to all during hot weather or with exercise. Dr. Wolff and others showed that the enlarged blood vessels were excessively permeable and allowed certain biochemicals to leak out and cause inflammation around the blood vessel wall. It was these irritating stimuli that caused the headache.

In the 1960s, cerebral-blood-flow studies showed that blood flow in the cerebral cortex (the outer layer of the brain) decreased during the migraine aura. This finding supported the narrowing or spasm of brain blood vessels as the cause of aura. But during the 1970s and 1980s, more sophisticated research revealed that the observed decrease in blood flow was usually insufficient to account for the disruption of brain function and the aura of migraine. It was more likely, the investigators concluded, that the decrease in cerebral blood flow during the aura was due to the decreased metabolic demand of nerve cells whose activity had decreased. The depression of nerve cell activity during the aura as well as the symptoms associated with the headache—for example, gastrointestinal disturbances and hypersensitivity to light—could best be explained by a primary disturbance of certain parts of the brain.

Nervous System Factors

The study of migraine has been hampered, of course, by the inability of researchers to directly examine the living brain of patients. While investigations of the electrical and, most recently, magnetic activities of the brain are limited in humans, a great deal of information has been obtained from studies of animal brains and the reactivity of animal nervous systems, vascular systems, and biochemicals. From these studies, there is growing evidence that changes in the brain initiate the series of events that leads to the aura and the entire migraine syndrome.

The aura of migraine is now thought to be attributable to a spreading "wave of depression" in the brain. The term *depression* as used here refers to a reduced level of nerve cell activity in the cortex. When the surface of an animal's brain is experimentally stimulated at a specific point, the activity of the underlying nerve cells is diminished, or depressed. This depression spreads slowly, like a ripple on a quiet pond. The stimulus to the animal brain might be analogous to the effect produced by a migraine trigger in the human nervous system.

Whether the trigger is outside the body or within it, a signal is relayed to centers deep in the brain. These centers in turn set off signals to other parts of the brain; the signals to the cortex cause a wave of reduced nerve cell activity. Blood flow decreases in this area not because of vasoconstriction, but because the depressed nerve cells no longer require the usual amount of blood. Other signals dampen the pain mechanism of the brain. The result is the aura of classic migraine, during which the patient experiences visual or other neurological symptoms, but no pain.

After 20 to 30 minutes, the aura subsides and the headache begins. This phase is associated with swelling of the blood vessels of the scalp and head and, again, may be initiated by different signals from brain centers. Then the vascular events described earlier take over. An inflammatory reaction occurs around the now-dilated blood vessel walls, either due to seepage of biochemicals through the blood vessel walls or to the reaction of neurotransmitters secreted by nerve endings in the blood vessel walls. In turn, the inflammation serves as an irritant that stimulates the nerve endings of the trigeminal nerve, which carries the pain message from the head and the face to the brain.

Chemical Factors

The signals or impulses transmitted from one brain cell (*neuron*) to another, or from nerve cells to muscle cells of blood vessel walls, are carried by biochemicals known as neurotransmitters. The neurotransmitters serotonin and noradrenaline play important roles in relaying these impulses. During the headache phase of migraine, reduced levels of serotonin have been noted in the blood. When levels of serotonin are reduced, large blood vessels in the head may dilate. However, the current belief is that changes in the amount of serotonin circulating in the blood is a secondary reaction, not the main event. Researchers are paying more attention to the role that serotonin and noradrenaline play as chemical messengers between nerve cells in the brain in initiating migraine. Other chemical changes probably also play a role in the development and conclusion of a migraine attack.

During the headache phase, a number of chemical messengers transmit the pain of migraine. In particular, the biochemical known as *substance P* transmits the pain message from the trigeminal nerve endings around blood vessels. (Substance P plays an important role in the production of pain in other parts of the body as well.)

In summary, the present concept of migraine mechanisms begins with an inherently susceptible individual who reacts to one or more triggering factors. These triggers affect centers deep in the brain, which then relay impulses to the cerebral cortex. There, certain neurotransmitters affect nerve cells, initiating the aura of migraine. After 20 or 30 minutes, other impulses from the brain release biochemicals that cause vasodilation and the sequence of events that leads to inflammation around the blood vessel wall. This inflammation constitutes the pain stimulus that is carried by the trigeminal nerve to the brain, where pain is experienced.

Classic and common migraine attacks probably have similar mechanisms. It is thought that in common migraine, the changes in the nervous system and the chemical changes that occur during the early part of an attack are insufficient to cause an aura. Some researchers, however, have suggested that common and classic attacks may involve two different events.

Research continues into exactly what happens in the brain during attacks of migraine.

TREATMENT

The ultimate goal of research into the mechanism of migraine is to help alleviate pain and discomfort. The term *cure* implies permanent eradication of the underlying cause of an illness. Unfortunately, there is no cure for migraine, nor is it likely that there will ever be a single treatment that is equally effective for all patients. But now migraine can be successfully treated. While ideal success would mean the suppression of all attacks, most migraine sufferers welcome any safe and acceptable treatment that reduces the number, severity, and duration of their attacks so they can lead normal lives. Today, migraine treatment is effective in as many as 80 percent of patients. What follows shows the wide range of available treatments.

Nondrug Treatments

Once your doctor has diagnosed migraine, you can take a number of steps on your own to reduce the stress and pain it causes.

- Give your physician a detailed and accurate medical history. This is important not only for a proper diagnosis but also to determine if any medications you might be taking for other conditions could be related to your migraine attacks. Similarly, the doctor will attempt to identify any other elements in your life that may be acting as migraine triggers.
- Learn how to cope with stress. You may decide to consult with a psychotherapist, use relaxation therapy (including meditation or biofeedback), try physical measures such as aerobic exercises, or enlist a combination of these or other pain-coping techniques (see chapter 5). Stress management can often significantly reduce the frequency and severity of your migraine attacks.
- Find and eliminate or control the factors that seem to trigger or aggravate your attacks. For example, you can change your diet to avoid the foods and beverages that seem to be associated with the onset of your migraines. Similarly, if you eat and sleep regularly and avoid long delays between meals, you may often reduce the incidence of attacks.
- During a migraine attack, seek out a quiet, dark room

where you can lie down without being disturbed. Apply an ice pack to the head; sometimes alternating cold and hot applications is useful. Vigorous massage of the temple on the side with the headache may also help, as may sustained pressure on the pulsing blood vessels at the temple. Try drinking small amounts of water or a thin soup to prevent dehydration.

A number of other nondrug approaches have been tried as treatments for migraine, with variable success. Some patients are helped by hypnotherapy, acupuncture, or transcutaneous electrical stimulation (TENS). These techniques are not for everyone, however, and usually don't produce lasting results.

The family and friends of those who experience migraine must be helped to realize that headaches are a very real and potentially debilitating condition that requires understanding and sympathy from those who are closest to the sufferer. During an acute attack, most migraine sufferers will want to withdraw from social activities. It's important for family members or others to allow them to do so, and not burden them with guilt—for missing a party or another social event, for example. Migraineurs will not want to engage in conversation, but will need to rest and be relieved as fully as possible of responsibility and outside stimulation. The help and protection of family and friends during these difficult periods is important to the migraine sufferer's sense of well-being.

Medications

There are two approaches to managing migraine headaches with medicine: the treatment of each acute attack, and the prevention of recurring attacks. Treating an acute attack means that at the first signs of onset the patient takes specific medication to ward off or reduce the migraine symptoms. Preventive therapy requires the patient to take an antimigraine drug every day to ward off repeated episodes.

Some medications can be used for both purposes, but because the doses used and the aims of treatment are different, each approach to migraine therapy is described separately here.

The treatment of an acute attack. In using drug therapy to treat an acute attack, medication is taken to stop the migraine in its tracks, before the attack fully develops. In addition to prescription drugs specifically aimed at halting the headache mechanism, antinausea drugs and painkillers are often used.

Ergotamine tartrate. This is the drug most commonly used to stop a migraine attack as it begins. Ergotamine tartrate is a vasoconstrictor that has been used against migraine for more than 50 years. It is effective in more than 80 percent of patients if taken during the first hour of either a classic or common migraine attack. In fact, the sooner the medication is taken, the greater the chance of putting an end to the attack.

How ergotamine tartrate works to relieve migraine is still uncertain. We know that it acts to constrict blood vessels that are in the process of swelling, but it may also have an effect on serotonin, and may act on the centers in the brain that are responsible for initiating the migraine attack.

Ergotamine tartrate is usually taken by mouth or as a rectal suppository, and it can also be taken sublingually (under the tongue) (Ergostat, Ergomar), by inhalation (Medihaler ergotamine), or by injection (DHE 45). Caffeine is often added to ergotamine tartrate, as in the brand-name substances Cafergot or Wigraine. The injectable form of ergotamine known as DHE 45 (dihydroergotamine) is usually reserved for patients with prolonged or severe migraine.

Like all medications, ergotamine tartrate can cause side effects, even when used properly. These effects *may* include nausea or vomiting, muscle aches, tingling of the extremities, chest pain, and a feeling of nervousness or tension. However, only about 10 percent of people who use ergotamine tartrate experience any of these side effects. Other medications that have similar actions—isometheptene mucate in the form of Midrin for example—may be prescribed in its place.

Ergotamine tartrate should not be used during pregnancy (it may induce abortion) or by people with high blood pressure, heart disease, vascular disease of the legs, or other vascular problems. It is not recommended for patients over 60 years of age because they are relatively more prone to vascular disease. Vasoconstrictors should not be used by patients with impaired circulation.

Caffeine. Many people with migraine have found that they feel better after consuming caffeine in a cup of coffee or a cola drink, and this alkaloid is often used for the treatment of acute migraine, usually in combination with ergotamine tartrate (Cafergot or Wigraine). Caffeine improves the absorption of other medications and enhances pain relief.

Antinausea drugs. During the acute attack, many migraine sufferers find that nausea and vomiting are as troublesome or even more disturbing than the headache. Moreover, ergotamine tartrate may worsen these symptoms. For this reason, an antinausea drug is often prescribed to be taken before any other medication. Metoclopramide (Reglan) helps to stop or reduce nausea and vomiting. Similar medications include: trimethobenzamide (Tigan), hydroxyzine (Vistaril), thiethylperazine (Torecan), promethazine (Phenergan), chlorpromazine (Thorazine), and prochlorperazine (Compazine).

Analgesics. If the headache is not fully stopped by the preceding medications, an analgesic (pain reliever) is often advisable. The pain reliever may be taken in addition to the above, or some people find relief by using only analgesics. Three over-the-counter varieties are available (aspirin, acetaminophen, and ibuprofen), packaged in many combinations, with or without other agents. If over-the-counter pain relievers are inadequate, your doctor can prescribe more powerful medications, chiefly the so-called nonsteroidal anti-inflammatory analgesics (NSAIAs) such as naproxen (Naprosyn) or many others (see page 68). These medications are often prescribed for arthritis and other painful conditions. Acetaminophen with codeine (Tylenol #3) may also be prescribed, or a combination of pain relievers, such as Fiorinal (aspirin, butalbital, caffeine) or Norgesic (aspirin, caffeine, orphenadrine citrate).

Caution: All of the analgesics (except the NSAIAs), caffeine, and ergotamine tartrate may perpetuate headaches on a rebound basis if they are taken every day or almost every day. *Never take these medications daily over a substantial period of time.* If you are taking analgesics on a regular basis and you are still bothered by headaches, you may be experiencing rebound headaches or a more serious problem. Consult your physician.

Treating the aura is usually unnecessary. However, the aura of classical migraine is sometimes unusually severe and may be more distressing than the subsequent headache. Agents that dilate blood vessels may abort the aura; these drugs include sublingual nitroglycerin and carbon dioxide. A popular remedy is breathing into a paper bag to build up carbon dioxide in the bloodstream. Remember, however, that these vasodilators may aggravate or trigger the headache phase of migraine.

Preventive medications. If your migraines occur two or three times a month or more, or if they are incapacitating and are not diminished or controlled by the medications recommended for acute attacks, your doctor may prescribe daily medication *to prevent* further attacks. Many of these daily medications have potentially harmful side effects and you must see your doctor periodically to monitor your progress.

Beta blockers. The most commonly used preventive medication is propranolol (Inderal), a drug originally developed for the treatment of high blood pressure and heart disease. Propranolol belongs to a class of drugs known as *beta blockers*, substances that block the impulses between certain nerve and muscle cells within the blood vessel walls. They counteract adrenaline-like reactions and thus lower blood pressure and heart rate. Propranolol is specifically approved by the Food and Drug Administration (FDA) for use in migraine, but other beta blockers, such as nadolol (Corgard), are also effective. The most common side effects of this class of drugs are fatigue, weakness, and cold extremities. A large drop in blood pressure or pulse may cause dizziness, fainting, and, in extreme cases, heart failure. These medications should not be taken by patients with asthma or certain heart conditions, and they should be used with caution by those with diabetes or thyroid disease.

Calcium channel blockers. These drugs are also used for heart disease and high blood pressure, and they have proved useful for preventing migraine attacks. (The term *calcium channel* has nothing to do with the calcium in bones, but with the flow of calcium ions into and out of tissue cells.) Calcium channel blockers, such as verapamil (Calan, Isoptin), probably act by stabilizing the tone of blood vessels and preventing the excessive changes in the size of blood vessels associated with migraine. The most common side effect of verapamil is constipation. These medications should not be taken by patients with certain heart conditions.

Antidepressants. Many of the medications that originally came on the market as antidepressants have been found to act in the nervous system to diminish pain, and they are now considered to be centrally acting analgesics. Among the most commonly used are amitriptyline (Elavil, Endep), doxepin (Sinequan, Adapin), and nortriptyline (Pamelor, Aventyl). The *potential* side effects are extensive, but the most common are dry mouth, drowsiness, and weight gain. These medications should be used with caution by patients with heart disease or glaucoma. Occasionally, other types of antidepressants are used, such as the monoamine oxidase (MAO) inhibitors (for example, phenelzine [Nardil]).

Nonsteroidal anti-inflammatory analgesics (NSAIAs). These drugs, such as naproxen (Naprosyn) or meclofenamate (Meclomen), not only may stop the pain of the acute migraine attack but, when taken daily, may also prevent attacks. They must be taken with food, for they often irritate the stomach, causing indigestion or ulcers.

Ergotamine tartrate. In addition to its value in treating acute attacks, ergotamine tartrate in small dosage (as in Bellergal) and similar medications, such as ergonovine, are also useful in preventing migraine attacks.

Antiserotonin agents. Methysergide maleate (Sansert) counteracts the effects of serotonin and is a very powerful migraine preventive. Methysergide is the only drug, other than propranolol, that is approved by the FDA for the prevention of migraine. Its main drawback is its ability to cause fibrous scar tissue in the abdomen, lungs, or heart when taken for an extended period of time. For that reason, it should never be used for more than six months without a break of one month. Methysergide should never be used in treating migraine attacks in children.

Cyproheptadine (Periactin) has some antiserotonin effects as well as functioning as an antihistamine. It has few side effects (mainly sedation) and therefore is often used to treat migraine in children.

A General Perspective on Drugs for Migraine

All of the medications for preventing migraine must be used under your doctor's supervision. Only the most common side effects have been listed here, but every medication has many *potential* side effects. It should also be noted that only rarely are these effects serious, and they almost always disappear with discontinuation of the medication. They do not affect the majority of patients to any major extent. Of course, if you notice any suspicious symptoms when taking any medication, consult your physician.

Unfortunately, the medications used to prevent migraine do not have a standard effect on every patient. For reasons that are not well understood, some patients react well to one medicine but not to another. Doctors start with the medicine or medicines that are most likely to work for the majority of people, but you may find that you have to try other medications on a trial-and-error basis.

Just as there is no uniformly effective medication, so, too, there is no standard dose. Common errors, made by both doctors and patients, are not sticking with a given medication long enough and using too small a dose. For example, 60mg of propranolol a day may prevent migraine in some patients; others may require 160mg, and a few others a much higher dose. Similarly, some patients find early relief with verapamil, but others find that

41

migraine episodes are not prevented until they have taken the medication for six weeks. Therefore, it is generally recommended that the dose of a migraine-preventive medication be slowly increased until effectiveness is noted, or until undesirable side effects require reducing the dose or substituting another medication.

New agents. The new drugs currently in development that show the most promise in the treatment of migraine are those that affect the action of serotonin. One such agent not yet on the market is sumatriptan, which increases the activity of serotonin and is used to abort an acute attack, presumably by constricting those blood vessels in the head that dilate during migraine. Unlike ergotamine tartrate, sumatriptan does not appear to constrict blood vessels in other parts of the body. Nevertheless, before they are allowed to become generally available, all new medications must first be proven safe and effective. They also must be experimentally compared with currently available and well-established drugs. Even if new products survive the many years between their initial development and their approval for use by patients, they may not be necessarily better than older, well-established ones.

THE TREATMENT OF EXCEPTIONALLY SEVERE MIGRAINE

If the medication you are taking is ineffective, and your migraine attack is so severe that you seek help, either in a doctor's office or a hospital emergency room, a physician usually administers an injection to abort the attack. The injection often contains a narcotic such as meperidine (Demerol) and a major tranquilizer and antinauseant such as hydroxyzine (Vistaril) or prochlorperazine (Compazine). Many specialists prefer to inject dihydroergotamine (DHE 45) and the antinauseant metoclopramide (Reglan). DHE 45, administered by injection, has a very rapid effect in halting a migraine attack. Metoclopramide is used to counteract the nausea and vomiting associated with acute migraine that may be aggravated by DHE 45.

Certain types of migraine attacks always require a doctor's attention. One is status migrainosus, which occurs when an extremely severe attack lasts for more than three days without relief. Hospitalization may be required to stop the attack, and intravenous fluids are often necessary to replace the fluid and minerals lost by vomiting. In such cases, dihydroergotamine is administered intravenously, along with an antinauseant. Potent painkillers, including morphine or meperidine, are sometimes needed to alleviate the severe pain, and major tranquilizers, such as prochlorperazine, are helpful. Corticosteroids also have proved to be useful in these cases.

When the headache is excruciating and cannot be alleviated by the usual means, many patients may fear they are undergoing a fatal attack. It is important that both physician and family provide the utmost in psychological support.

On rare occasions, visual loss, weakness or numbness on one side of the body, or other neurological symptoms that constitute the aura of classic migraine, may last for days or become permanent. Very severe migraine can lead to a stroke— migrainous infarction. Fortunately, this complication is extremely rare.

ARE YOU SURE IT'S MIGRAINE?

As we have noted, the diagnosis of migraine is based on the medical history, not on the examination of the patient or on laboratory tests. Sometimes the characteristics of the headache may lead the patient, the physician, or both to wrongly consider it migraine. The following case illustrates this point:

Joyce L., a 25-year-old teacher, awoke one morning with a throbbing pain in the left temple. The pain did not respond to aspirin, and she felt vaguely ill, but she had no other symptoms. Because the pain grew more intense, she went to the emergency room at a nearby hospital. The results of her general physical examination and neurological examination were normal. Questioning determined that both Joyce's mother and sister had experienced migraine attacks, which were at their worst during menstruation. Joyce had begun to menstruate just prior to her attack, and the combination of these factors led her and her physician to agree on the diagnosis of migraine. She was given an injection of meperidine (Demerol), and soon the pain had subsided to a great degree.

Joyce went home, but after a few hours the pain increased again. She took aspirin and was able to fall asleep. The following morning, the pain was severe again. She returned to the emergency room and was told that a migraine attack can last for two days; she was given another meperidine injection, and again the pain was alleviated, only to return again several hours later.

On the morning of the third day, Joyce awoke with throbbing pain in the left temple, but now the pain extended into her mouth, above the left upper molar. In addition, there was swelling of the gum and some swelling of the face. She went to her dentist, who quickly found an abscessed tooth. The abscess was drained, and she was given an antibiotic. Her headache disappeared that night.

As this case history demonstrates, not all one-sided throbbing headaches are migraine—even if there is a strong family history of migraine and, as in this case, the headache is coincident with menstruation. This patient did not experience the typical nausea or intolerance to light or noise that almost invariably accompanies migraine. As we have observed, migraine is a difficult diagnosis to make on the basis of a single attack. The first attack of one-sided headache may indeed be migraine, but the symptom may be the result of a number of other conditions. In this case, it was caused by an infected tooth; in other cases, more serious diseases might be discovered. It is, therefore, particularly important that your doctor rule out any underlying organic disease before considering the diagnosis of migraine (see chapter 7).

MIGRAINE SYMPTOMS

Common Migraine

- The attack may be preceded by prodromal symptoms (such as drowsiness or restlessness) several hours or a day before the headache.
- The headache is most often located on one side, usually around the temple.
- Quality of pain: typically throbbing or pulsating.
- Degree of pain: moderate to severe.
- Duration: several hours to three days.
- Frequency: from rare and occasional to several per week; average is one to three episodes per month.
- Symptoms accompanying the headache include nausea, hypersensitivity to light and sound, and potentially many other disturbances such as dizziness and agitation or depression.
- Common triggering factors include menstruation, relaxation after emotional stress, changes in sleeping or eating patterns, high humidity, rapid changes in the weather,

alcohol, and certain foods. Physical activity usually aggravates the headache.

Classic Migraine
- Defined by the presence of the aura (visual or other neurological disturbances) that precedes the headache by 20–30 minutes.
- Headache features, as well as prodromal and associated symptoms, resemble those of common migraine but need not be as well defined.

TREATMENT

For Acute Attacks
- Ergotamine tartrate preparations (often including caffeine [Cafergot, Wygraine]).
- Antinausea drugs (metoclopramide [Reglan], promethazine [Phenergan]).
- Analgesics (over-the-counter: aspirin, acetaminophen [Tylenol], ibuprofen [Advil, Nuprin]; prescription: naproxen [Naprosyn], indomethacin [Indocin], codeine).

Preventive Therapy
- Beta blockers (for example, propranolol [Inderal]).
- Antidepressant analgesics (for example, amitriptyline [Elavil]).
- Calcium channel blockers (for example, verapamil [Calan, Isoptin]).
- Nonsteroidal anti-inflammatory analgesics (NSAIAs) (for example, naproxen [Naprosyn]).
- Vasoconstrictors (for example, small doses of ergotamine [Bellergal]).

- Antiserotonin agents (for example, methysergide maleate [Sansert]).

Nondrug Techniques
- Elimination of migraine triggers.
- Relaxation techniques.
- Learning to cope with stress.

(These are useful to both diminish and prevent attacks.)

2

Tension Headaches

The headaches that most of us experience from time to time are commonly called *tension headaches*. The International Headache Society, a group of doctors who have expertise in the field of headaches, uses the term *tension-type headache* to indicate how uncertain researchers are about the mechanism of these headaches. The headaches are not necessarily related to psychological or muscle tension. Although tension headaches also have been referred to as *muscle-contraction headaches*, it is a term that, as we shall see, is also somewhat misleading.

Tension headaches comprise approximately 60 percent of all headaches that are not related to an underlying disease. Most people who experience *occasional tension headaches* don't bother to consult a physician, and for the most part medical help isn't required. The pain is usually mild to moderate, with a sensation of tightness or pressure across the forehead, on both sides of the head, at the back of the neck, or even extending to the shoulders. In most instances, the headache soon disappears, either by itself or with the help of over-the-counter pain relievers. Almost everyone has experienced such occasional headaches, and they are not a cause for concern.

However, chronic headaches recurring on a regular basis pose a more serious problem—one that is likely to (or at least should) lead the sufferer to seek medical help. Some patients report having headaches characterized by a steady ache or pressure on both sides of the head every day, or almost every day, for months or even years. These recurring or constant tension headaches are referred to as *chronic daily headaches*, and require medical attention.

OCCASIONAL TENSION HEADACHES

Symptoms

The pain of tension headache is usually described as a mild or moderate dull ache, or a feeling of pressure, often reported as resembling a bandlike feeling of tightness around the head or a tight "cap" on top of the head. People often experience the sensation as discomfort rather than actual pain. The headache usually occurs on both sides of the head, either at the front or back, and sometimes extends into the neck or shoulders. This is not always the case, however; some people have tension headaches that occur on one side only or are scattered over different parts of the head. Indeed, there is no single standard pain location for those who report these headaches.

Frequency and duration. As their name implies, occasional tension headaches usually don't occur with regularity, nor do they interfere with the sufferer's daily activities. If they are noted once a week or more, they may be evolving into the chronic form.

Tension headaches may last an hour or two, all day, or longer. An individual acute attack often occurs in late afternoon or evening, when the stresses of the day have built up.

Associated symptoms. Unlike migraine, tension headaches are not characteristically associated with symptoms other than pain or discomfort in the head. Sometimes, however, minor symptoms, similar to but less prominent than those seen with migraine, may occur. Some people might experience a degree of sensitivity to light, sound, or odors. Sometimes even slight nausea or, more often, a decrease in appetite may be present.

Causes

Psychological factors. There is no one factor that causes occasional tension headaches, nor is there a ready list of triggers, as in the case of migraine. Individuals vary widely in their tendency to get these headaches. Some people report that their headaches are associated with psychological stress, such as job interviews or family disagreements. A headache may appear before, during, or after a stressful event; for many people, they occur as an occasional reaction to the normal stresses of everyday life. Emotional factors are more clearly associated with chronic daily headaches than with occasional tension headaches.

The case of Maria S. is an example of an occasional tension headache that appears to be associated with everyday stresses.

Maria is a 14-year-old girl whose family had recently moved to a new city. Her headaches began a few months before her visit to the headache clinic; they roughly coincided with the beginning of her first year of high school. She described the headaches as a tight sensation around or over the entire head, as though she were wearing a hat that was too tight. The pain was not severe, but was sufficiently disturbing that she had difficulty concentrating in school. On two or three occasions, the school nurse sent her home after she had complained of a headache.

Each of Maria's headaches would last for several hours or all day. First they occurred only occasionally, then two or three times a week. Maria was especially sensitive to noise during a headache, and she didn't want to talk or interact with other people while a headache was in progress. Features of migraine, such as throbbing pain, nausea, and oversensitivity to light, were absent. When questioned, at first she reported no aggravating or triggering factors. Aspirin or acetaminophen afforded incomplete relief. Neurological and physical examinations were normal, and the diagnosis of tension headache was made.

After seeing her physician on several occasions, Maria became more open and discussed her apprehension about starting high school. She was a better than average student, but she was afraid that she would not do well. She described several of her teachers as "too tough" and not understanding, and said she hadn't made any new friends in school. These problems were discussed with Maria's parents, who in turn discussed them with her teachers. Maria was reassured with regard to the quality of her work. She became more confident and began to make friends. Nothing other than occasional use of over-the-counter medication was recommended. The headaches gradually disappeared over the next six months and did not recur.

Physical factors. While emotional components may play a role in tension headaches, the pain is definitely not imaginary; it involves very real changes in the body.

We noted earlier that in the past many physicians referred to tension headache as "muscle-contraction headache." For years it was thought that the main physical mechanism behind these headaches was an overcontraction or tensing of the scalp, neck, and related muscles. For example, in some people jaw clenching was thought to play a role in initiating headaches. However, a number of studies over the last fifteen years have shown that the tensing of the scalp and face muscles is not *consistently* related to the occurrence of tension headaches. Measurements of the degree of muscle contraction can be made and recorded as an electromyogram (EMG). EMG studies have shown as much muscle activity in the scalp of patients with migraine headaches as in those with tension headaches. If and when excessive muscle tensing does occur, it may simply *contribute* to the pain of a headache.

What is the physical cause of tension headaches? The answer isn't simple, nor is it fully known. Muscle activity is initiated by chemical reactions, which it also produces. Some biochemicals are toxic, and they would cause pain if they weren't carried away by the bloodstream. When there is a buildup of toxic biochemicals during physical activity, muscles become painful. A common example is a muscle cramp that strikes during exercise. Such pain occurs when muscle contraction is so intense that the toxins accumulate faster than they can be cleared away by the bloodstream, or when the blood supply is inadequate for the needs of normal muscle activity—for example, when there is spasm of the arteries. Both mechanisms have been implicated in the pain of tension headaches. Another common theory holds that conscious or unconscious emotional stress causes excessive muscle contractions that in turn lead to pain.

Head pain also has been shown to occur when the scalp muscles are exercised while deprived of blood. In one such experiment, a tight band was placed around the head to shut off muscle blood supply, and the subject was asked to chew continuously, which involves using the muscles over the temples. Pain quickly occurred. But if vasoconstriction were the sole mechanism involved in causing head pain, then alcohol, a vasodilator, might be expected to relieve the headache—just the opposite of the situation in migraine. While alcohol might indeed bring temporary relief, a couple of drinks may inadvertently make a headache worse. Fortunately or unfortunately, liquor does not have a consistent effect when taken for tension headaches. Most probably, no single physical mechanism is at work in these headaches.

Tension headaches, both occasional and chronic, can also occur in migraine sufferers, either between migraine attacks (*interval headaches*) or mixed with bouts of migraine (*mixed headaches*). Moreover, as migraine attacks increase in frequency, they tend to lose the characteristics of migraine and take on the features of tension headache, finally evolving into *chronic daily headaches*.

Recent studies have shown other relationships between tension headaches and migraine. Patients with both tension headaches and migraine have lower blood levels of the neurotransmitter serotonin than people who don't suffer from these headaches. Migraine and tension headache sufferers have lower cerebrospinal fluid levels of endorphins, chemicals in the nervous system that decrease the perceived intensity of pain. Whether decreased levels of these important brain chemicals help to explain attacks of tension headache, migraine, or both is the subject of ongoing research. In any case, these findings have led many researchers to believe that migraine and tension headache share a common mechanism centered in the brain.

Examination

If you are subject to recurrent headaches, your physician must first make sure that no underlying illness is causing your pain. Most headaches caused by an underlying disease become worse with time, or are associated with other telltale symptoms or signs that help to differentiate them from other forms of head pain.

Medical examinations usually find physical signs to be normal in people who experience tension headaches. However, muscles at the temple or on other parts of the head or neck may be tense or tender. Your doctor also may discover *trigger points* in the muscles of your scalp, neck, or face. Exerting pressure on these tiny knots of muscle causes pain; the pain may be located at the point of compression, or the compression may bring on the customary pattern of tension headache at a distance from the trigger point.

Certain tests can determine to what degree you may be physically—as opposed to emotionally—tense, suggesting that your headaches have a physical component. For example, a clue that a headache is a tension headache is the general inability to physically relax. Your physician lifts your arm, tells you to imagine that you are relaxing in an armchair, and then withdraws his support. The ordinary reaction is for the arm to drop loosely, involuntarily; however, many people are so tense that once the support is removed they keep their arms poised in the air. Similarly, jaw clenching is another sign of physical tension. Your doctor may grasp your jaw to determine how easily it can be moved, or feel your jaw muscles to estimate the degree of tension.

Because relaxation therapy is one of the main ways of treating tension headaches, it is important to determine whether your headaches have a physical component. Part of the therapy involves your becoming aware of the role played by this physical tension and precisely how it can contribute to your headaches.

While certain features of the physical examination may reveal tightness (*spasm*) or tenderness of muscles, or a general difficulty in relaxing, these findings are by no means either dramatic or inevitable in people who experience tension headaches. This inconsistency is the reason why physicians still debate the underlying mechanism of the condition.

Treatment

When most people get a single acute tension headache, they either let it run its brief course or use one of the commonly available over-the-counter pain relievers. These are either aspirin, acetaminophen, and ibuprofen, sometimes used in combination with other ingredients, such as caffeine. (The chart on pages 67–69 lists some of the most commonly used formulations.) If tension headaches begin to occur frequently, biofeedback or other relaxation techniques can help, too (see chapter 5).

If, however, you are experiencing frequent tension headaches and aren't getting sufficient relief from over-the-counter products, or if you are taking pain relievers for headaches more often than twice a week, it's time to consult a physician.

CHRONIC DAILY HEADACHES

Many people experience the symptoms of tension headache every day, for months or years. Headaches of this frequency are termed *chronic tension headaches* or *chronic daily headaches*. They have the same characteristics as occasional tension headaches—the pain is dull and aching in quality and mild to moderate in severity, and affects various parts of the head. The headaches may last for several hours or all day, from morning until night, and they occur every day, or almost every day. As we noted previously, these chronic daily headaches can often evolve from previous migraine attacks, and they are often associated with the overuse of medication.

Rebound Headache:
A Major Cause of Chronic Daily Headache

The medications that line the shelves of pharmacies and super-markets across the country are effective for the great majority of occasional tension headaches. They are less useful for treating chronic—that is, frequently recurring or daily—headaches, and they may even perpetuate your pain. Unfortunately, many patients consume increasing amounts of these medications, sometimes at their physicians' direction, with the hope of finding relief. This is a dangerous practice, for several reasons.

The case of Lorna R. is a typical example of the problems encountered with medicating chronic daily headaches.

The patient is a 35-year-old accountant whose headaches have been constant for the previous six years. In her twenties, she suffered from occasional one-sided, throbbing headaches that were accompanied by nausea or loss of appetite and intolerance to light. These frequently coincided with her menstrual period or occurred after a stressful event. The pain was usually of moderate severity, but sometimes it was disabling. She did not consult a physician for these headaches; over-the-counter medication relieved her pain slightly.

In her late twenties, the headaches began to increase in frequency to several times a month. Lorna consulted a doctor, who prescribed medication consisting of acetaminophen, a barbiturate, and caffeine. This treatment alleviated her headaches considerably, but did not decrease the frequency of their occurrence. As time went on, the medication seemed to be decreasing in effectiveness, and she switched to over-the-counter pills. Soon she began to take two tablets instead of one, and then three tablets instead of two, and to use the medication every other day instead of once or twice a week. Eventually, she found herself taking about a dozen tablets every day because the pain had become daily and continuous.

As her use of medication escalated, the pattern of her headaches changed. Instead of being confined to one side, they now occurred over the back or front of her head or were scattered over different areas. They had an aching quality, and although they were much more frequent, they were also less severe. Lorna no longer experienced nausea or other symptoms, as she had with her one-sided headaches. She could function during a headache, but they interfered with her ability to enjoy life and to relate to her family and friends. There seemed to be no obvious triggering factors, although it appeared that emotional stress made the headaches worse. She denied experiencing depression or any change in her personality, but her husband reported that she had lost interest in outside activities, preferred not to socialize, and that her sex drive had disappeared.

Neurological and general physical examinations were normal. The patient's expression was not particularly sad, but it was lacking in spontaneity.

At first Lorna said that she was now taking no medication for her headaches, but by the end of the examination she admitted that she was taking approximately 12 tablets of an over-the-counter pain reliever every day. This consisted of a combination of aspirin, acetaminophen, and caffeine. She neglected to mention this painkiller, rationalizing that "medication is something that's prescribed by a doctor, not something you buy in a grocery store." The diagnosis was chronic tension headache (chronic daily headache).

Although each dose of the medicine brought her little relief, Lorna was afraid to give up her over-the-counter pain medication. She was reassured that other medications would be prescribed for her headaches, and she was instructed on how to taper her current dosages, taking fewer and fewer tablets each day over a period of several weeks. A nonsteroidal anti-inflammatory (NSAIA) pain reliever was prescribed instead of the combination of aspirin, acetaminophen, and caffeine. In addition, a tricyclic antidepressant was prescribed.

Once Lorna had stopped taking her daily, habitual medication, the headaches markedly diminished, both in frequency and intensity. Within a month, she was back to her normal self. She occasionally had recurrences of the headaches, but these were easily countered with prescription nonsteroidal anti-inflammatory pain medication, and the headaches no longer interfered with her life. In time, she was able to taper off and discontinue the use of the substitute drugs as well.

The headaches this patient had experienced in her twenties had been migraines, although they were not diagnosed by a physician at the time. As is so often the case, when the migraine attacks increased in frequency, they lost their migraine characteristics and evolved into daily tension headaches.

Many patients with chronic daily headaches take excessive amounts of over-the-counter or prescription pain relievers, and this overuse may exacerbate headaches on a rebound basis. In Lorna R., the medication had become a trigger rather than a treatment for headache. As the level of the medication in the blood drops (hours after one has taken it), the mechanism causing the pain, briefly suppressed by the medication, rebounds, producing a "new" headache or exacerbating the residual headache. The natural tendency is to take more and more pills, at shorter and shorter intervals. For a period of time this strategy "works" in that the head pain is partially or completely controlled. But as the medication becomes less effective, the headaches rebound with increasing frequency, finally recurring daily and lasting virtually all day. Thus, many people end up taking dozens of pills a day, inadvertently feeding the fire they are trying to extinguish.

This strategy is not only counterproductive, it is actually dangerous. Every medication, including common over-the-counter products, has potential side effects. Acetaminophen, for instance, taken in high doses for long periods of time, may cause damage to the liver. Aspirin and ibuprofen can upset the stomach and cause gastritis or ulcers; these medications may also injure the kidneys. All of these side effects are more likely to occur in a more severe form if there is underlying disease or dysfunction of the liver, stomach, or kidneys.

Caffeine, included in some of the combination pain-relief formulations, is useful for the short term; it enhances the effect of aspirin and acetaminophen. In the long run, however, caffeine, whether in pain medications or in coffee, tea, or soft drinks, can cause rebound headaches, anxiety, jitteriness, palpitations, and other adverse effects.

Prescription medications for headache can have a similar effect. Aspirin and acetaminophen may be prescribed in combination with a barbiturate (as in Fiorinal or Fioricet, for example) or in combination with codeine or a codeine-like product (for example, Synalgos or Percocet). These prescription drugs are more powerful than the over-the-counter pain relievers and, because of the barbiturates or narcotics they contain, are more habit-forming and thus more easily abused. Prescription barbiturates and narcotics can produce physical dependence. Barbiturate or narcotic withdrawal, for example, may be accompanied by serious side effects, including sweating, agitation, palpitations, and seizures.

Abruptly discontinuing any of these medications may trigger severe headaches and, sometimes, other problems. Gradual withdrawal is therefore necessary. The NSAIA pain relievers temporarily prescribed for Lorna act at the site of pain, while the prescribed antidepressants block pain in the central nervous system. Neither of these types of medicine causes rebound headaches.

It cannot be stressed too strongly that pain medications designed to be taken for an occasional acute headache can do considerable harm when taken daily, or almost every day.

Emotional Factors in Chronic Daily Headaches

For patients who experience tension headaches almost every day, emotional factors almost always play a role. It may be difficult to determine, however, whether psychological factors such as depression and anxiety are a cause of stress and headaches or their consequence. Some headache patients who appear depressed and have lost interest in their family and friends will nevertheless deny feelings of sadness. Others will assert that their only problem is the headache, that they feel "down" because they are in pain, and that if only the pain were to disappear, their lives would be perfect.

Physicians will sometimes debate this issue with their patients in an effort to convince them that emotional factors are the root cause of their headaches, but this is a circular argument that serves no constructive purpose. Depression can make pain worse, and pain can cause depression. The truth is that after years of suffering daily or almost daily headaches, it doesn't matter which came first. What *is* important is to acknowledge that both the pain and the patient's response to it (the two cannot really be separated) must be addressed if the patient's quality of life is to be improved. Without attempting to determine which came first, the emotion or the physical pain, let us now examine the psychological factors in chronic daily headache.

Depression. A large proportion of patients who suffer from chronic headaches show signs of depression. The depression may not be obvious to the headache sufferer or even to his or her family, friends, or associates. Depression typically involves symptoms like feeling sad or "down" much of the time, as well as feelings of helplessness and low self-esteem. Physical symptoms, such as difficulty in falling asleep or staying asleep, may also be present. Some people report feeling fatigued or "blue" upon awakening. Some suffer a loss of appetite or, conversely, may eat excessively. Constipation or other gastrointestinal symptoms may also occur. Loss of sexual desire is a very common symptom of underlying depression. People who are depressed may feel listless and have difficulty concentrating, and, in some cases, experience memory impairment. In mid- or late life, depression may even be mistaken for Alzheimer's disease.

In some patients, headaches may occur as a form of "masked depression." According to one line of psychiatric thinking, the experience of head pain may be an unconscious substitute for psychic pain. When this occurs, patients may not be aware of their depression. Although this circumstance is rare, it nevertheless constitutes an important condition.

In studies of patients with chronic tension headaches, the most common emotional factors noted were depression and repressed anger toward family members or superiors at work. Sexual problems in marriage also were common and were frequently linked to long-term resentment toward a spouse. Interestingly, one study found that depression and anxiety were present in 95 percent of patients with tension headaches, as opposed to 54 percent who had migraines.

Stress and anxiety. Anxiety is common in those who suffer chronic headaches. Such people often complain of feeling tense, uneasy, "uptight," seemingly without obvious cause. Anxiety also tends to lower the pain threshold and frequently accompanies depression.

Whether we realize it or not, most of us live complicated lives. The demands made on us by family, friends, employers, and fellow workers are complicated by the demands we make on ourselves and the major and minor annoyances of everyday life— all of which have the potential to cause intense stress. Our emotional and physical reaction to stress depends not only on the circumstances that we encounter on a daily basis, but also on the way we deal with them. Getting stuck in traffic on a quiet afternoon will provoke quite a different reaction to delays experienced while going to a job interview. Individual vulnerability is important. Stress can trigger a philosophical resignation in one person, a headache in another, or an asthma attack in a third.

Many people who experience chronic tension headaches also suffer from various forms of anxiety and unresolved emotional conflicts. The irony is that at least some of the patient's repressed anger, frustration, or hostility may be a response to unsympathetic co-workers, friends, or family members who view the chronic headaches as a character flaw. Sometimes anger and hostility are legitimately directed at a physician who has advised, "The headaches won't kill you. Learn to live with them," or at a doctor who gives you only a few moments of his or her time, seeming to pay more attention to patients who are more easily treated or who have "more important" conditions.

Tension headaches, both occasional and chronic, usually have meaning in the life of the sufferer. For example, if you get a headache when you're faced with a conflict, you may be subconsciously transferring an emotional conflict into a physical one; the headache may serve as a form of psychological defense. In the middle of an argument, a headache provides you with a very good reason for ending the argument right then and there. ("I can't talk about this now. I have a headache.") It's important for all of us who may suffer from headaches to consider their meaning in our lives and to ask ourselves what purpose they may be serving. The simplest way to do this is to consider under what circumstances

the headaches occur and to determine whether there is any particular social or emotional pattern to their occurrence.

Treatment of Chronic Daily Headaches

Medications. Are there any pain medications that can safely be
taken for chronic daily headaches? As the preceding case history
indicates, two types of medication are available for this purpose.
One acts by inhibiting the chemicals in the body that initiate the
pain at the site where it is experienced (for example, in the
muscles). The other type acts in the brain and spinal cord to block
the pathways that lead to the brain's perception of pain. Most
common pain relievers act at the periphery—that is, at the site
where the pain is felt.

The pain relievers that act at the site of pain include the
nonsteroidal anti-inflammatory analgesics (NSAIAs), which are
not usually associated with rebound effect. Ibuprofen, which is
sold over the counter, is a member of this family of drugs, and
there are more than a dozen others that may be obtained by
prescription. These include naproxen (Naprosyn), meclofenamate sodium (Meclomen), piroxicam (Feldene), ketoprofen
(Orudis), and indomethacin sodium trihydrate (Indocin), among
others. The NSAIAs act against inflammation and pain, but,
unlike cortisone or other steroids, they do not have a steroid
chemical base. The most common side effects seen with the
NSAIAs are gastrointestinal distress, including bleeding peptic
ulcers. If you have had these conditions or kidney disease in the
past, you should inform your physician and take these drugs with
extreme caution, if at all.

As we noted in discussing migraine, it has been determined
that some medications created to treat depression also relieve pain
by their action in the central nervous system—that is, in the brain

and the spinal cord—and that this analgesic action is unrelated to their antidepressant effects. These tricyclic antidepressants are very useful in treating chronic, frequently recurring, or daily tension headaches. Not only do they decrease pain, but they may also relieve depression (the pain-relieving dosage is usually lower than the antidepressant dose). Remember, however, that you don't have to be suffering from depression to get pain relief from these drugs. Their most common potential side effects are dryness of the mouth, constipation, drowsiness, and some weight gain. They should be used with caution by people with heart disease, chronic urinary problems, or glaucoma.

Of the other medications that block pain centrally, codeine, morphine, and meperidine (Demerol) are the most widely known. Because these drugs are addictive, and often have to be administered in ever increasing doses, they are not recommended for benign, frequently recurring pain, including migraine or tension headache.

Since there is often a close association between migraine and chronic daily headaches, those medications used to prevent migraine may also be useful in treating chronic daily headaches. These include the beta blocker propranolol (Inderal) and the calcium channel blocker verapamil (Calan, Isoptin). The side effects most commonly encountered with propranolol are fatigue, weakness, and cold extremities; if pulse and blood pressure drop too low, lightheadedness and fainting may occur. Propranolol should not be taken by patients with asthma or certain heart conditions, and it should be used with caution by those with diabetes or thyroid disease. The most common side effect of verapamil is constipation. It, too, should be used with caution by patients with certain heart conditions.

If your headache is due to tense muscles, why not treat it with a muscle relaxant? Unfortunately, there isn't a good muscle relaxant that can be taken orally without causing a great deal of drowsiness. Tranquilizers such as diazepam (Valium), oxazepam (Serax), and alprazolam (Xanax) may be useful, but taken chronically they are potentially habituating, and must therefore be used only with considerable caution.

Relaxation techniques. Of the several nondrug treatments that have been successful in alleviating pain, the most important with regard to tension headaches are relaxation exercises, especially biofeedback techniques. Once your doctor has explained the role of emotional stress and physical tension in triggering tension headaches, the idea of performing special exercises to help you relax may not seem quite so exotic. In fact, learning to relax may do more to help curtail or prevent your headaches than many of the standard medications. (These exercises and other techniques are described in chapter 5.)

One series of exercises involves a pattern of contracting and then relaxing different sets of muscles. Other relaxation techniques include listening to special relaxation tapes, and applying the practices of transcendental meditation. All of these methods have proved effective in helping to reduce the frequency or severity of different kinds of headaches, especially tension headaches. Biofeedback techniques, which enable people to monitor their own physical responses, are some of the best methods for inducing a relaxation response (see page 119).

Many habitual postures of standing and sitting or other activities can cause muscle strain or tension, and these have been identified as primary causes of chronic headaches. Becoming aware of such behavior, as well as understanding how generally to reduce the physical tension you may be expending in your daily activities, can be effective in preventing or managing tension headaches.

Relaxation techniques used alone may not totally eliminate your headaches. While it is usually necessary to supplement relaxation with prescription medication, their value as a treatment mode should not be underestimated.

Psychological management. Whether consciously or subconsciously, people often feel that their chronic headaches are a reflection of their personalities—their headaches are "proof" that they can't handle the stressful situations that others seem to manage quite well. From this perspective, the headaches may become an excuse for unsatisfactory performance, and initiate an entire syndrome in which individual strengths and liabilities become narrowly evaluated within a framework dominated by the presence of headaches. Such a perspective is not uncommon, so it needs to be emphasized that tension headaches are not necessarily related to a *specific* stressful event; they may simply be the body's reaction to the many accumulated stresses of everyday life. This kind of basic psychological understanding is crucial to headache management. (The psychological aspects of headache management are explored in detail in chapter 5.)

Outlook

While it is unrealistic to expect a complete cessation of your tension headaches, the goal of treatment is to decrease the frequency and severity of the episodes so that an occasional headache can be overcome with medication or relaxation techniques, or a combination of both. The result of successful treatment should be a return to a normal life so that your headaches no longer interfere with work or pleasure.

THE CHARACTERISTICS OF TENSION HEADACHE

- The headache is most often located on both sides of the head, or as a bandlike sensation around the head.
- Quality of pain: typically dull, aching, an unpleasant tightness.
- Degree of pain: mild to moderate.
- Duration: one hour to all day.
- Frequency: occasional tension headache can occur twice a week to once a month or less; chronic tension headache can occur daily or almost daily.
- Associated symptoms: none or mild.
- Underlying factors: migraine, overuse of pain medication, muscle tension, emotional stress, depression, anxiety.

TREATMENT

Medication for Occasional Tension Headaches
(not to be taken more than twice a week)

Over-the-counter pain relievers
- aspirin (Empirin, Bufferin)
- acetaminophen (Tylenol, Datril)
- ibuprofen (Nuprin, Advil)
- aspirin + caffeine (Anacin)
- aspirin + acetaminophen + caffeine (Excedrin)

Prescription pain relievers
- aspirin, caffeine, barbiturate (Fiorinal)
- acetaminophen, caffeine, barbiturate (Fioricet, Esgic)

- aspirin and orphenadrine (Norgesic)
- acetaminophen and codeine (Tylenol with codeine)
- acetaminophen and hydrocodone (Vicodin)
- acetaminophen and oxycodone (Percocet)
- propoxyphene (Darvon)

Nonsteroidal anti-inflammatory analgesics (NSAIAs) (all by prescription only, except ibuprofen, which is available over the counter)
- diclofenac (Voltaren)
- fenoprofen (Nalfon)
- flurbiprofen (Ansaid)
- ibuprofen (Advil, Medipren, Nuprin, Motrin)
- indomethacin (Indocin)
- ketoprofen (Orudis)
- meclofenamate (Meclomen)
- mefenamic acid (Ponstel)
- naproxen (Naprosyn)
- naproxen sodium (Anaprox)
- piroxicam (Feldene)
- sulindac (Clinoril)
- tolmetin (Tolectin)

Medication for Chronic Daily (Tension) Headaches
For headache prevention:

Tricyclic antidepressants/pain relievers
- amitriptyline (Elavil)
- desipramine (Norpramin)
- doxepin (Sinequan)
- imipramine (Tofranil)
- nortriptyline (Pamelor)
- protriptyline (Vivactil)

- trazodone (Desyrel)*
- trimipramine (Surmontil)

NSAIAs (see listing above)

Medications employed to prevent migraine that may also be useful:
- propranolol (Inderal)
- verapamil (Calan)

Nondrug Therapies for Both Occasional and Chronic Tension Headaches
- Gradual withdrawal from daily medications designed for acute occasional pain.
- Avoidance of triggering factors.
- Relaxation techniques.
- Attention to emotional factors.

*Not a tricyclic

3

Cluster
Headaches

The cluster headache is one of the most painful of all medical conditions, and certainly the most painful of headaches. Its specific characteristics are in sharp contrast to both migraine and tension headaches. For one thing, approximately 85 percent of all cluster headache sufferers are men, a reverse of the situation with migraine and tension headaches. And the pain of cluster headache is truly excruciating. Sufferers have been known to bang their heads against the wall in an effort to relieve their pain, and some have committed suicide. Normal life for sufferers of cluster headaches may become virtually impossible during a series of attacks, known as the *cluster period*.

Fortunately, the cluster headache is far less common than migraine or tension headache. Considerably less than 1 percent of the population has experienced bouts of this disturbing type of headache, probably between 500,000 and 1 million people in the United States.

In the past, the cluster headache was referred to as "Horton's headache" and "Harris's neuralgia," named after the physicians who studied the disorder in the United States and England, respectively. In Europe, the cluster headache is still often referred to as migrainous neuralgia. This term is somewhat misleading, for although both migraine and cluster headaches involve vascular mechanisms, there are important differences between the two conditions. Nevertheless, some people are unfortunate enough to suffer from both migraine and cluster headaches, or a combination of the two.

SYMPTOMS

The pain of cluster headaches is variously reported as sharp, piercing, boring in the drilling sense, or, less often, as throbbing. It impels people to move about, rock, or even, as noted, to hit their heads against the wall. The headaches are recurrent and always appear on one side of the head, usually around the eye, temple, or forehead; sometimes, the pain may begin in the neck or other areas of the head. For most sufferers, the pain always recurs on the same side of the head. This is in contrast to migraine, which may affect right or left sides on different occasions. Cluster headache sufferers do not experience any warning sign, such as the prodrome or aura that may occur with migraine. The cluster headache can occur at any time of day or night, but interruption of sleep by a painful attack is common. In fact, cluster headaches most often occur at night, during rapid eye movement (REM) sleep. This segment of the sleep cycle takes place approximately every 90 minutes and is characteristically associated with dreaming.

Symptoms that usually accompany this fierce headache include tearing or redness of the eye, stuffiness or running of the nose, as well as a drooping eyelid, all on the side with the headache. A narrowing of the pupil may accompany the drooping eyelid, and facial sweating may also be present.

The cluster headache derives its name from the fact that the attacks occur in series or clusters. Single episodes usually last from 20 minutes to 2 hours; occasionally, residual discomfort may last for several hours. Typically, the sufferer experiences one to as many as five attacks a day, every day, for weeks or months. In the most common form, *episodic cluster headache*, the attacks will spontaneously disappear after a number of weeks or months, only to return with a vengeance weeks, months, or a year or more later.

AGE AND GENDER

Cluster headaches most often first occur between the ages of 20 and 40; however, they can appear at any age. Rare cases of very young children (some as young as three years old) who appeared to suffer from cluster headaches have been reported in the medical literature. As we noted earlier, cluster headaches, unlike migraine or tension headaches, are far more prevalent among men than among women.

VARIETIES OF CLUSTER HEADACHES

The type of cluster attack just described is known as *episodic cluster headache*, and the majority of cluster headache patients (approximately 80 percent) fit into this category. They experience periods of daily headaches lasting weeks or months, and then are free from further episodes for extended periods—weeks, months, or years. During the *susceptible cluster period*, drinking alcohol usually will initiate a cluster headache; however, during the period of remission, most sufferers can use alcohol in moderation without fear of setting off an attack.

Some unfortunate individuals, however, are unrelentingly susceptible to attacks. Rather than experiencing periods of remission that alternate with periods of cluster headaches, they experience one or more daily attacks without any extended period of relief. This pattern of recurring headaches is known as *chronic cluster headache*. The term *chronic* may be slightly misleading in that it could also apply to the recurrent periods of episodic cluster headaches, but this isn't the case. People with chronic cluster headaches experience the same headaches described above, with the same accompanying symptoms. The difference is that, unlike episodic cluster headache patients, they don't have the benefit of weeks or months during which they are free of attacks. There are two subdivisions of chronic cluster headaches: (1) chronic cluster headaches that are unremitting from onset; and (2) chronic cluster headaches that evolve from episodic cluster headaches.

A rare form of cluster headache is *chronic paroxysmal hemicrania*. These headaches are similar to the attacks described earlier, but they are much briefer in duration, lasting only a few minutes, and they occur many times a day. In fact, patients with this condition have reported experiencing up to a dozen or more attacks in a single day. Unlike the typical forms of cluster headaches, chronic paroxysmal hemicrania is seen mostly in women. Fortunately, this form of cluster headache responds well to a specific medication, indomethacin sodium trihydrate.

On rare occasions, the features of cluster headache may be mixed with attacks of migraine (*cluster-migraine syndrome*) or with trigeminal neuralgia/tic douloureaux (*cluster-tic syndrome*).

TRIGGERS

Drinking alcoholic beverages is by far the most common trigger of an attack of cluster headache if the patient is in a cluster period. Since the reason for this lies in alcohol's action as a vasodilator, it makes sense that other substances that dilate blood vessels can also trigger the headaches. These include foods that contain nitrites, such as hot dogs or smoked meats, as well as certain medications such as nitroglycerin, used to treat heart disease and high blood pressure. (Again, it's important to tell your doctor *all* the medications you may be taking, even those for conditions that are unrelated to your headaches.) As we have noted, cluster headaches often occur during REM sleep. The reasons for this are unknown, but this stage of sleep seems to act as a triggering factor.

Interestingly, in studies that have looked at the habits of people with cluster headaches, it was found that as many as 91 percent drank alcoholic beverages regularly and nearly two-thirds classified themselves as "heavy" drinkers. These patients usually don't have to be told not to drink during a cluster period, since the relationship between alcohol and an attack is obvious. What's more, as many as 94 percent of sufferers were smokers. Many smoked heavily—the average was a pack and a half of cigarettes a day.

Unlike migraine or tension headache attacks, cluster headaches are not triggered by emotionally stressful incidents in daily life. While migraine and tension headaches can occur either during or directly after a stressful incident, no such pattern has been observed for cluster headaches.

During the periods when they are susceptible to attacks, people with cluster headaches have an understandable tendency toward depression and anxiety, as well as sleep disturbances. Rather than triggering the headaches, the depression and anxiety probably are the result of the recurrent and very painful daily attacks.

PHYSICAL AND PERSONALITY CHARACTERISTICS

One researcher in the field of cluster headaches, Dr. John R. Graham, found a number of characteristics shared by many men with cluster headaches. He described cluster sufferers as "leonine" or having a lionlike facial appearance with furrowed brows. His description of a "typical" cluster headache patient also includes large body type, ruddy complexion, thick orange-peel-like facial skin, and a generally stoical expression. The psychological prototype is that of a hardworking, somewhat passive male who rarely expresses his feelings. As with migraine sufferers, psychological profiles are by no means invariable.

In any case, the pain of a cluster attack is usually so excruciating that even some of the strongest and most stoical men will cry out in agony during an episode, weeping or screaming with pain. Many pace the floor and others run out of the house in their distress. Lying still and resting seems to make the cluster headache worse—just the opposite of migraine. Most sufferers shut out their families or whomever else might be around, and become totally noncommunicative. It must be emphasized that such uncharacteristic behavior is based not on hysteria, but on an all-too-real physical pain.

UNDERLYING MECHANISMS

In the medical literature, cluster headache is classified as a form of vascular headache, as is migraine. Nevertheless, the precise role of the changes in blood vessels that take place during an attack is still a matter for investigation. In a sense, cluster headache is more of an enigma than either migraine or tension headaches. Only rarely has there been a pattern of family inheritance for cluster headache patients, for example. Furthermore, researchers have yet to discover exactly why the headaches occur in clusters or why they disappear for an extended period before returning. There is, however, general agreement that this sequencing is caused by a disturbance in the part of the brain known as the hypothalamus—the center for the "biological clocks" that direct our normal body rhythms, such as sleeping, eating, and hormone regulation.

Research has shown that blood flow in some extracranial vessels (blood vessels in the head but outside the brain) increases significantly during a cluster attack. With the increased blood flow and associated vasodilation, the skin temperature on the side of the head with the headache often increases by 1° to 3° C. This temperature increase is particularly apparent around the eye, temple, and cheek.

The vascular role in cluster headache is substantiated by the fact that attacks can be initiated or made worse by drinking an alcoholic beverage or by absorbing another vasodilator, such as nitroglycerin or histamine. Moreover, attacks may be stopped with ergotamine tartrate and prevented with methysergide, two medications that are vasoconstrictors and thus tend to reverse blood vessel dilation.

It is thought that certain hormones play an important role in cluster headache, as well as in migraine. Abnormalities in the rhythmic secretion of several hormones have been found during the cluster period. Moreover, levels of the male sex hormone, testosterone, are decreased in men during the periods when they have cluster attacks, compared with levels in the same men during periods of remission. The marked sex distribution of cluster and migraine patients, with 85 percent of cluster patients male and 75 percent of migraine patients female further implicates the sex hormones.

Exactly what hormonal or other chemical changes in the body control the timing of attacks is not known, but it is the subject of extensive study. If researchers could discover what changes initiate the period of remission from attacks, it might be possible to find a way to prevent cluster attacks altogether.

DIFFICULTIES IN DIAGNOSIS

Cluster headache is usually easily differentiated from migraine or tension headache by its clearly discernible characteristics, yet errors in diagnosis continue to occur. They usually relate to the misinterpretation of the pain and associated symptoms. The very intense pain is often attributed to a suspected underlying physical problem (a brain tumor, for example). The associated clogged and draining nostril is frequently misdiagnosed as sinus disease. The tearing and reddened eye may be falsely attributed to an allergy. Because physicians so often mistake these symptoms, it is especially important for you to describe them clearly, and to be specific about the timing of the attacks. In particular, it is the periodic nature of cluster attacks that helps to determine the correct diagnosis.

The case of James H. provides an example of how cluster headache patients can go for years without being correctly diagnosed or treated.

The patient, a 26-year-old bond salesman, had experienced severe headaches on and off for the past six years. A severe boring-like pain would appear between his right eye and nose and would radiate above and below the eye, in the area of the sinuses. At the same time, he noted nasal clogging and a discharge from the nostril, as well as tearing of the eye. He assumed that this condition had something to do with sinusitis and consulted an ear, nose, and throat specialist, who agreed with that diagnosis. Although the physician could find no evidence of disease, he treated James H. with medication for sinusitis. The medication had no immediate effect, but the headaches disappeared after another month.

The next year, in the spring, the same type of headaches returned. This time James H. was referred to an allergist. Numerous allergy tests were performed, and the patient was found to be allergic to certain molds and dust. He then underwent a course of desensitization, and after a month or two, he assumed the treatment was successful because the headaches disappeared. This general sequence of events occurred every year for six years. During that time, James H. also sought treatment from other ear, nose, and throat specialists and allergists. Then, by chance, he read about cluster headaches in a popular magazine, and the description seemed to fit his headache pattern.

Indeed, when he visited the headache unit, he was found to exhibit all the characteristics of cluster headache. He had a severe, boring pain in and around one eye that lasted for several hours and occurred once or twice every day, sometimes awakening him from sleep. During an attack, he could not lie down but felt impelled to pace back and forth. The redness and tearing of the eye and clogging and drainage from the nostril on the side with the headache were also typical symptoms. James H. was a heavy smoker and noted that in the spring, when the cluster of attacks occurred, he could not drink alcohol without bringing on a headache. Finally, after six years of painful, recurrent headaches, the correct diagnosis of cluster headache was established. Appropriate therapy helped to prevent further attacks.

TREATMENT

Cluster attacks are intensely painful and disruptive, but there are a variety of available treatments that offer relief. As with other types of headaches, treatment includes both the termination of an acute attack and therapy to prevent further attacks. Because cluster headaches recur daily, treatment to prevent subsequent attacks plays as great a role as treatment for an acute single headache.

The first advice is to stop drinking alcoholic beverages and to stop smoking cigarettes. While the relationship between cluster headaches and cigarette smoking is unclear, the fact that over 90 percent of people with cluster headaches smoke does suggest a strong association. Preventing the vasodilation associated with alcohol helps right away; stopping smoking, on the other hand, often does not result in an immediate obvious benefit, but may over the long term.

Nonpharmacologic therapies such as relaxation techniques and psychological counseling have proved effective in treating migraine and tension headache. Unfortunately, these and similar nondrug treatments have not been successful in reducing either the severity or the recurrence of cluster headaches. Thus, with the exception of oxygen administration (see page 80), the emphasis here will be on treating the condition with medication.

During an attack, there is relatively little that family members or friends can do for a cluster headache sufferer other than to be sympathetic. They should not urge the patient to lie down, since doing so actually makes the pain worse. Probably the best thing one can do is to convince the sufferer to consult a physician if he or she has not already done so or is, for some reason, hesitant to do so.

Treatment of Acute Attacks

Ergotamine tartrate. The standard treatment for a single *acute* attack of cluster headache is the vasoconstricting drug ergotamine tartrate, the same prescription medication that is used to treat migraine attacks. As in migraine, ergotamine tartrate must be taken at the very first sign of a headache to halt the attack effectively. Because a cluster headache begins quickly and lasts a relatively short period of time, getting the ergotamine tartrate into the bloodstream quickly is essential. Ergotamine tartrate administered by inhalation or placed under the tongue is more rapidly absorbed than when taken by mouth. In some cases, cluster patients are taught to give themselves the injectable form of ergotamine, known as DHE 45. When used as directed, it has proved to relieve or curtail cluster attacks in as many as 70 percent of patients.

Side effects that may occur with ergotamine in all its forms include nausea or vomiting, muscle ache, tingling of the extremities, chest pain, and a feeling of tension. However, only about 10 percent of patients experience some of these symptoms. As we noted earlier, you should not take ergotamine if you have high blood pressure, heart disease, or vascular disease of the legs. It should not be prescribed during pregnancy and is usually not prescribed for people over 60 years of age because of its vaso-constricting effects.

Administration of 100 percent oxygen. One nondrug therapy that has proved very effective in shortening individual acute episodes of cluster headache is the administration of 100 percent oxygen. Usually inhalation through an oxygen mask at a high flow rate for 5 to 15 minutes will abort the attack. Of course, this treatment requires supervision by your doctor and involves your having an oxygen tank or canister and mask available for home or office use. Oxygen therapy has proved effective in relieving symptoms in as many as 80 percent of patients.

Local anesthetic. The nerve impulses that set off the mechanism of cluster headache pass through a structure called the sphenopalatine ganglion. This is a nerve relay station that is located at the base of the skull, underneath the mucous membrane that lines the back of the nose. The sphenopalatine ganglion can be blocked with a local anesthetic, intercepting the nerve impulses that trigger the headache. For optimal effectiveness, the anesthetic must be applied at the end of a probe that is then passed deep into the nose. Obviously, running to a doctor's office to get this treatment when an attack is in progress is highly impractical, but nose drops containing lidocaine or similar anesthetic agents can be self-administered and are sometimes effective.

Analgesics. Commercially available over-the-counter painkillers usually do little or nothing to relieve cluster headache pain. Narcotics, although sometimes effective, are not usually prescribed because of the dangers of potential overuse; however, your physician may prescribe narcotic analgesics if other treatments are contraindicated or have not been effective.

PREVENTIVE TREATMENT

While ergotamine tartrate and oxygen offer relief from single attacks, they don't solve the cluster headache patient's real problem: the recurrence of attacks. If you experience episodic cluster headaches, chronic cluster headaches, or chronic paroxysmal hemicrania, you probably suffer with these headaches virtually every day. Given this oppressive reality, the main goal of any approach to treatment must be to prevent your headaches from recurring. Fortunately, a variety of medications have proved to be effective as *preventive* therapy.

Ergotamine tartrate. If attacks regularly occur at a specific time—for example, at the same time every night—physicians may prescribe ergotamine tartrate in *anticipation* of the attack. Ideally, in order to ward off cluster attacks, ergotamine must be taken within the two hours *before* the predicted attack. Sometimes it is prescribed to be taken three times daily as a strategy to prevent attacks. Because this exceeds the safe dosage, patients must be closely watched for signs of ergot toxicity. These include nausea or vomiting, muscle aches, tingling, burning, or numbness of the hands or feet, and chest pain.

Prednisone. This drug is a corticosteroid that has proved to be effective in preventing cluster headaches. In one study, 76 percent of patients had their attacks fully prevented with prednisone, and 12 percent showed partial improvement. Prednisone works quickly in preventing attacks and its use can often be stopped after 7 to 10 days when it is usually administered along with verapamil or methysergide.

Potential side effects of long-term prednisone treatment are numerous. They may include reduced immunity against infection, gastric ulcers, weight gain, worsening of high blood pressure or diabetes, and personality changes. For people who experience these problems, prednisone should be taken with caution or not at all.

Calcium channel blockers. Usually used to treat heart disease and high blood pressure as well as for preventive therapy in migraine, these medications, especially verapamil (Isoptin, Calan), have recently proved useful in preventing cluster headaches. Calcium channel blockers reach their maximum effectiveness slowly—after several weeks—and may have to be used in much higher than standard dosages for effectively preventing the cluster headache syndrome. The most common side effect is constipation. These agents should not be used by patients with certain heart conditions.

Methysergide maleate (Sansert). While methysergide maleate is often used with great success as preventive therapy, it should not be taken daily for periods longer than six months; otherwise potentially serious side effects, including the development of fibrous scar tissue in the body, may develop. Since most bouts of episodic cluster headaches are shorter than six months in duration, methysergide can be taken during such a period in relatively high doses, with little danger of serious side effects. It successfully prevents attacks in some 70 percent of patients.

Lithium carbonate. The fact that prednisone and methysergide maleate cannot be used for extended periods of time without potential serious side effects is particularly unfortunate for patients with chronic cluster headaches that persist without remission. A medication that has been especially useful for this condition is lithium carbonate (Eskalith, Lithane, Lithobid), an agent commonly used in the treatment of manic depressive attacks. Precisely how lithium works to prevent chronic cluster headaches is not known, but it appears to affect the biological cycles controlled by the hypothalamus. It is disruptions in these cycles that can trigger such periodic diseases as manic depression and cluster headache. Lithium is particularly useful for chronic cluster headaches, but may also be used for episodic cluster headaches.

Lithium carbonate may cause a number of side effects. Early, but usually transient, symptoms include trembling and gastrointestinal disturbances. Toxic levels of lithium are associated with abnormal movements, confusion, and even coma. If lithium is prescribed for you, your doctor will periodically want to measure the amount of the drug present in your blood in order to make sure it is not above the level considered safe. This careful monitoring is indispensable. Patients taking lithium should use diuretics only with caution, because these agents may elevate lithium blood levels.

Other medications. A number of other medications that may be prescribed to help prevent cluster attacks include beta blockers, such as propranolol (Inderal); tricyclic antidepressants, such as amitriptyline (Elavil); major tranquilizers, such as chlorpromazine (Thorazine); monoamine oxidase (MAO) inhibitors, such as phenelzine (Nardil); nonsteroidal anti-inflammatory agents (NSAIAs), such as indomethacin (Indocin); and anticonvulsants such as divalproex (Depakote). Sometimes these medications are combined with one of the agents listed earlier.

All these medications have potential side effects and are not prescribed for people with certain concomitant conditions. Again, the importance of providing your physician with a complete medical history, as well as a list of all the medications you may be taking, cannot be overemphasized. Don't depend on the physician to elicit this information from you; be prepared to volunteer it, and to see that it's taken into account.

Treatment for Chronic Paroxysmal Hemicrania

This variation of cluster headache predominantly affects women and occurs in the form of many brief attacks a day. The drug that has proved most effective in treating chronic paroxysmal hemicrania is indomethacin (Indocin). Indeed, if the headaches do not respond to this medication, the diagnosis must be doubted. Like other NSAIAs, indomethacin may irritate the stomach, causing indigestion or ulcers. It must therefore be taken with food.

If None of the Standard Treatments Work

Sometimes, all the available medications fail to prevent cluster headaches. More extreme measures must then be pursued. *Blocking the occipital nerve* with a local anesthetic and a steroid agent is sometimes helpful. This is accomplished by a relatively simple injection into the back of the scalp, but the effect is often incomplete and only temporary.

Because blood levels of the chemical histamine are raised during an attack of cluster headache, *histamine desensitization* was touted by Dr. Bayard Horton of the Mayo Clinic many years ago. When other physicians could not duplicate his reports of success, the treatment fell into disrepute. But intravenous histamine therapy, administered while the patient is hospitalized, was resurrected several years ago. It has been effective in about a third of the cases in which it has been tried.

As a last resort, surgery may be necessary. Because the pain of cluster headache is carried along the trigeminal nerve deep in the face, injuring this nerve by means of *radiofrequency coagulation* will usually prevent the painful attacks. However, permanent loss of sensation in the forehead and the eye also results; in the latter case, the eye may be predisposed to recurrent inflammation.

OUTLOOK

If you or someone close to you suffers from this very painful condition, it's important to realize that many different treatments are available, and the chances are that one of them will be successful. At this stage of our understanding of the condition, there is no reason for anyone to suffer the agony of recurring attacks of cluster headaches.

THE CHARACTERISTICS OF CLUSTER HEADACHE

- The headache is always located on one side of the head, in and around the eye, temple, or forehead.
- Quality of pain: burning, boring, sharp, or throbbing.
- Degree of pain: very severe, excruciating.
- Duration: 20 minutes to 2 hours.
- Frequency: one to six times per day, for several weeks or months; often awakens patient from sleep.

- Associated symptoms: redness and tearing of eye, stuffiness and drainage of nostril, drooping eyelid—all on the side of the headache.
- Aggravating factors: alcohol and other substances that dilate the blood vessels.
- Course: clusters of daily headaches usually disappear after weeks or months, but may return months or a year later. (The chronic form has no pain-free periods.)

TREATMENT

Treatment of single acute attack of cluster headache
- ergotamine tartrate (Ergostat, Medihaler ergotamine)
- inhalation of 100 percent oxygen
- sphenopalatine ganglion block.

Prevention of episodic cluster attacks
- ergotamine tartrate (Cafergot)
- prednisone (Deltasone)
- calcium channel blockers (verapamil [Calan, Isoptin])
- methysergide maleate (Sansert)
- lithium carbonate (Eskalith, Lithane, Lithobid)
- Medications employed to prevent migraine that may also be useful: beta blockers (propranolol), tricyclic antidepressants (amitriptyline), and NSAIAs (indomethacin).

Surgery
- Radiofrequency coagulation of trigeminal nerve

Prevention of chronic paroxysmal hemicrania
- Indomethacin sodium trihydrate (Indocin)

4

Headache Triggers

As we have seen, a great many ordinary matters—stress, certain foods—can trigger headaches of varying scope and intensity in susceptible individuals. Since so many of these factors can also initiate a headache in people who don't habitually suffer from migraine, tension, or cluster headaches, a closer look at them is in order.

Certain headaches are not only triggered by emotional factors but constitute one of the major manifestations of a particular emotional condition; they are known as "psychogenic" headaches. Several other rather uncommon types of headaches are named after their triggering factors; they are usually of short duration.

Note: Your headaches may very well be related to one of the triggers described in this chapter, but what you think of as a headache trigger may be only a coincidental factor. If your headaches frequently recur, or are interfering with your daily activities, consult a physician. It's the doctor's role to first make sure that the headache isn't being caused by an injury or an underlying disease. Only when that is established can you be advised about the best way to treat your headaches and to prevent future ones.

TRIGGERS OF COMMON HEADACHES

Almost anything can trigger a headache, from everyday events and conditions in the environment to the internal changes that take place in our bodies. The environmental factors include the foods, beverages, and medications we consume as well as such external influences as industrial chemicals in the air or water and changes in the weather.

Foods and Beverages

Of the many environmental factors that may trigger headaches, foods and beverages are perhaps the most common. There is a long list of potential culprits, and for someone who is susceptible, almost any food or drink can precipitate migraine or another form of headache. On the other hand, only about 15 to 20 percent of people with migraine demonstrate a specific food sensitivity. (The term *food sensitivity* is not synonymous with *food allergy*. An allergy derives from a disturbance in the immune mechanism of the body, while a food sensitivity involves other changes in body chemistry that take place when a particular food is ingested.)

In most cases, no single agent is responsible for causing the headache, but rather a combination of biochemicals, natural or artificial, that act during a period of heightened susceptibility. Because of these variable factors, a piece of chocolate, for example, can trigger a headache at one time and not another. The dose of the triggering factor is important as well. While one piece of chocolate may not cause a headache, eating an entire box of chocolate might have a very different result.

Sometimes the relationship of a specific food to a subsequent headache is obvious because it's immediate and consistent—for example, migraine initiated as a reaction to alcohol use or chocolate binges. On other occasions, however, you may not be aware that a particular food is triggering your headache. In these circumstances, if medication and other treatments have failed, your doctor may eliminate one food after another from your diet in an attempt to isolate the offending item. A less time-consuming but draconian approach, rarely used, is to eliminate *all* food for a limited period of time and ingest nothing more than vitamins, minerals, and water. Foods are then reintroduced into your diet, one by one, to determine what food or food product will trigger a headache.

One way a food can trigger headaches is by dilating the blood vessels in the head. This reaction sets off a series of events identical with or similar to those seen in migraine headaches (see chapter 1). Alcohol and the nitrites in sausages and hot dogs can cause this sort of reaction, while other foods trigger headaches by causing more complex alterations in body chemistry. Many foods that contain proteins having an amine in their structure are implicated as triggers. Tyramine, which is found in many foods (hard cheeses, for example) is a frequent headache trigger, as are chocolate and some other foods that also contain phenylethylamine. The protein l'octopamine in citrus fruits is another potential triggering agent.

DIET FOR PATIENTS WITH MIGRAINE

GUIDELINES: This diet is best used in conjunction with a diary. If you get a headache, review the list of foods to avoid and record any that you may have eaten in the 24 hours prior to headache. After several headaches, review your diary to look for patterns. Once your headaches improve, you may introduce foods you like one at a time to see if your headaches get worse.

A dietary factor usually does not precipitate a headache every time and limits need not be absolute. Two factors are important:

1. The quantity of the food trigger: One bite of chocolate may not trigger a headache; eating a whole box is more likely to do so.
2. The interaction with other headache triggers: Drinking one glass of wine may not trigger a headache; wine combined with another trigger (such as cheese) or when imbibed under stress is more likely to do so.

FOODS	TO AVOID	ALLOWED
Beverages	*alcohol, *esp. red wine*	fruit juices
	caffeine—coffee, tea, cola drinks	††no more than 1 cup coffee, 2 cups tea, 2 soft drinks
	chocolate or cocoa	
		noncola soft drinks (ginger ale, club soda)
		decaffeinated drinks
Dairy products	milk, buttermilk, cream	milk with 1% or 2% fat, skimmed milk
	†sour cream	no more than ½ cup of yogurt
	ice cream	
	†yogurt	(only cottage and cream cheese with MAOI medication)
	hard (aged) cheeses, processed cheeses	††soft cheeses (except camembert, mozzarella, and brie)
		whipped cream
		butter, margarine
		cooking oils

FOODS	TO AVOID	ALLOWED
Meats	*processed meats:* hot dogs, sausage	fresh or frozen meats
	*aged, cured, or canned meats (ham, bacon)	
	meat pies	
	*beef liver	
Poultry	*chicken liver	fresh or frozen poultry
		no more than 3 eggs per week
Fish	**pickled herring*	fresh or frozen fish
	*dried smoked fish	canned tuna and salmon
Vegetables	*most beans	string beans
	onions	onions only for flavoring
	most peas	
	olives, pickles	asparagus, beets, carrots, spinach, tomatoes, squash, corn, zucchini, broccoli, lettuce
	sauerkraut	
		potatoes
Grains		rice, spaghetti and other pasta

FOODS	TO AVOID	ALLOWED
Breads and cereals	yeast breads (white breads), sourdough breads donuts, cakes most cookies	††whole wheat and rye breads English muffins, melba toast bagels, matzoh most cereals
Soups	soups containing MSG or yeast soups from bouillon cubes	homemade soups preferred to canned soups
Fruits	*citrus fruits, bananas,* figs, raisins, papaya, kiwi, plums, pineapples, †avocados	prunes, apples, cherries, grapes, apricots, peaches, pears
Desserts and snacks	*chocolates ice cream cookies/cakes made with yeast nuts, seeds peanut butter	fruits, as above sherbet Jello cookies/cakes made without yeast jam, jelly, honey sugar candy
Additives	*MSG* and other flavor enhancers (frozen TV dinners often contain MSG)	white vinegar salad dressing (in small amounts)

FOODS	TO AVOID	ALLOWED
Additives (*continued*)	artificial sweetener (NutraSweet)	artificial sweetener (Saccharin)
	meat tenderizers	
	†soy sauce	
	seasonings and spices	
	pizza and other mixed dishes	
	marinated foods	
	*yeast extracts	

*These items are to be particularly avoided by those people taking MAO (monoamine oxidase) inhibitor medication.

†These foods may be eaten with moderation.

††Allowed if restrictions are not severe.

Foods set in italics are the most common triggers of migraine.

Alcohol

Among foods and beverages, alcohol is probably the most common headache trigger. We noted earlier how alcohol, due to its vasodilating properties, can act as a potent trigger for those people who are susceptible to migraines or cluster headaches.

Almost everyone, at one time or another, has suffered the unpleasant experience of a *hangover headache*. Most of us have learned that the simplest way to avoid such a headache is to eat before and while we drink, and to drink in moderation and at a leisurely pace. Not everyone reacts to alcohol in the same way, though. Certain people may get a headache from even small amounts of alcohol—not hours after drinking, but almost immediately. They do so because they have a sensitivity to either the alcohol itself or to another ingredient in the drink—to what is usually referred to as a *congener.*

Congeners are what makes red wine taste different from white, and scotch different from cognac or vodka; they are either additives or ingredients of the material from which the beverage is made, including products of the distillation or aging process. Some of the more common congeners are fusel oil, esters, certain acids, tannins, and aldehydes.

Some people report that only one type of alcoholic beverage sets off their headaches. For the most part these are beverages that contain a high degree of congeners—red wine and bourbon are cited as particular offenders in this regard. Most red wines contain sulfites, so it's possible that some of these people are reacting to the sulfites rather than to the alcohol itself. (A number of states now require that wine labels include a warning about the presence of sulfites in a wine.)

Vodka, the alcoholic beverage that contains the lowest level of congeners, is associated with a smaller likelihood of hangover symptoms. Nevertheless, drink enough vodka and you'll get a headache. Both the alcoholic and the congener content of a drink help determine how bad a hangover you might have in the morning.

The contribution of congeners to hangover headaches is considered important, although the actual mechanism is unknown. A hangover headache cannot be attributed to the vasodilation induced by an alcoholic drink, because the alcohol has been metabolized by the body and the vasodilation has largely subsided by the time the headache occurs. Excessive alcoholic intake is often associated with dehydration, and this, too, may play a role in causing the hangover.

Many investigators suspect that a hangover headache acts in a way similar to that of the rebound headache caused by the overuse of certain medications. In other words, as the bodily changes induced by the alcoholic beverage dissipate, the body *reacts* with a headache and the other symptoms of the hangover syndrome. In support of this concept is the fact that another drink or two may temporarily diminish the headache and other features of the hangover—the "hair of the dog" theory. Needless to say, this practice is definitely *not* recommended. Not only can the headache return, but there is the danger of perpetuating and encouraging the alcohol habit, which can lead to even worse consequences. Consuming alcoholic beverages in excess is associated with liver failure and other severe medical and emotional problems. (Pregnant women should avoid drinking alcohol *in any amount*.)

It makes sense to abstain completely from alcohol if you find that a particular drink, or alcohol in any form, gives you a headache. If you do choose to drink moderately, always try to eat while drinking to help protect the stomach. Eating a snack before going to bed, honey on crackers or a fruit juice similarly high in fructose content, is also a good idea; the fructose may help to metabolize the chemical products of alcohol that tend to cause headaches and other hangover symptoms.

Food Additives

Monosodium glutamate (MSG). This flavor enhancer and tenderizer, commonly added to a variety of foods, is another dietary substance that can cause headaches in some people. The most famous example of reaction to MSG is the "Chinese restaurant syndrome," first reported in the 1960s. The MSG reaction occurs approximately 20 minutes after eating and may include sweating, a sense of burning and tingling of the face and chest, dizziness, and headache. Today, not all Chinese restaurants use MSG, and as people have become more health-conscious, many restaurants will prepare your dinner without it if you request that they do so.

Not everyone gets a headache when they eat foods or products that contain MSG. In fact, most people don't. But since MSG is of no known nutritional value, you may still want to avoid it, particularly since it is also a potential trigger in migraine sufferers. Although Chinese food is the most commonly cited culprit, many other foods contain MSG, especially those that are prepared or prepackaged, including a number of brands of instant and canned soups, TV dinners, processed meats, tenderizers and seasonings, and dry-roasted nuts. Look carefully at the labels when you purchase such products so you can avoid unpleasant reactions.

Spices. If you do get a headache after eating certain foods, it may not necessarily be from MSG. Spices used in some foods, particularly in Indian, Mexican, and other "hot" cuisines, have caused reactions, including headaches, in some people. Experience is your best guide here. If a certain favorite dish regularly gives you a headache, it's better to avoid it.

Nitrites. This additive is found in many foods, including hot dogs, corned beef, salami, sausage, bologna, bacon, and other aged meats. Nitrites are used to maintain the red color of these meats and they act as preservatives. They may be impossible to detect, as in the salads of some restaurants and retail stores. Nitrites may cause dilation of blood vessels in the head and trigger migraine. If you are susceptible to headaches, avoid foods that contain nitrites.

Aspartame (NutraSweet). This is a commonly used artificial sweetener. There is now some evidence that it may provoke migraine.

Natural Foods

Amines. This term refers to a family of proteins, many of which are essential to life because they cannot be manufactured by the body and must be obtained from the foods we eat. One of the essential amino acids that the body cannot manufacture is tyramine.

Paradoxically, a high intake of tyramine and other foods high in amine content may cause headaches, especially migraine, in susceptible individuals. Chocolate and citrus fruits, which contain complex amines (for example, phenylethylamine and l'octopamine) frequently trigger migraine attacks. Tyramine, the amine most frequently implicated in provoking migraine headaches, is an ingredient of many foods. (Studies have demonstrated that pure tyramine itself does not trigger migraines. Again, we must presume that there are additional agents or factors that combine with tyramine to act as a trigger.) Tyramine is found in alcoholic beverages (particularly red wine), dairy products (aged and hard cheeses), certain meats and fishes (cured or processed meats, liver, herring), yeast products (certain breads and fresh cake), fruits (figs and raisins), broad beans, and nuts. (See the chart on pages 89–93.)

Caffeine. An alkaloid found in coffee, tea, and many soft drinks, caffeine plays a double-edged role in headaches. Known to enhance the absorption of pain relievers, it even seems to possess some analgesic properties of its own. Thus, a strong cup of coffee may help alleviate a headache. As we noted earlier, it is sometimes added to many over-the-counter pain relievers and prescription medications that are used to treat a variety of headaches.

On the other hand, caffeine has been implicated as a trigger for two different kinds of headaches. The first is the type of headache that is triggered by a caffeine overdose or toxicity when you drink too many cups of coffee or other caffeine-containing beverages — for example, tea or some soft drinks. Other symptoms of caffeine excess may include stomach upset, insomnia, irritability, trembling, diarrhea, and dizziness. First aid for acute caffeine overdose includes drinking a considerable amount of water, lying down, and taking an over-the-counter analgesic for the headache. If you regularly get headaches or other symptoms that may be related to drinking too much coffee or other caffeine-containing beverages, the obvious answer is to stop drinking these beverages and to switch to decaffeinated versions.

The second kind of headache involving caffeine is caused by caffeine withdrawal. When cutting down on the amount of coffee you drink, do it gradually or your headaches may get worse as the result of the rebound effect noted earlier. In addition to this rebound headache, people who ingest increased amounts of caffeine are subject to a more subtle rebound reaction that is often difficult to recognize as such. This rebound headache reaction often occurs in people who drink many cups of coffee or caffeine-containing soft drinks in a day. As caffeine levels in the blood fluctuate, the decrease of caffeine in the blood triggers the headache mechanism that had been suppressed by the earlier higher blood levels of caffeine.

Some people may get both kinds of caffeine headaches. If they drink as many as 10 or more cups of coffee daily, they surpass the level of their caffeine tolerance and get a headache resulting from caffeine toxicity. At night, they refrain from coffee and sleep; in the morning, deprived of their customary intake, they have a headache from the overnight caffeine withdrawal. While these may seem extreme cases of caffeine "poisoning," it's worth remembering that caffeine is a powerful drug, and that ingested above certain levels, it is toxic. As is the case with any drug, the actual level of toxicity varies from person to person, depending on customary intake and individual tolerance. In addition to causing headache, abrupt withdrawal from the habitual use of caffeine may induce depression.

Because drinking large amounts of coffee has been implicated in other health problems—including increases in blood pressure and cholesterol levels and gastrointestinal problems—it makes sense to restrict your coffee intake to no more than two or three cups a day. Coffee contains about twice as much caffeine as tea or other caffeine-containing beverages (for example, cola drinks or cocoa); the exact amount varies from 85mg to 150mg per cup, depending on the way the coffee is brewed. Coffee lovers should know that the highest caffeine is found in brews made by using the drip method, somewhat lower amounts result from percolation, lower still is the amount found in instant coffee. Remember, too, that many pain medications (both over-the-counter and prescription) contain high doses of caffeine and may therefore cause all of the problems noted above.

MEDICATIONS AND DRUGS

As an unwanted side effect of their action, a variety of medications can initiate headaches. These drugs include nitroglycerin, which is often used to treat coronary heart disease. In recent years, nitroglycerin has been increasingly administered in the form of a timed-release patch that is worn on the skin. The result is that it is delivered to the system slowly throughout the day and night; this gradual action is less likely to cause headache than the quick action of a tablet taken under the tongue.

High blood pressure medications, especially the drugs reserpine and hydralazine, also are known to cause headaches. Contraceptive pills containing estrogens also may aggravate or trigger migraine and other headaches. The birth control pill is not absolutely forbidden for use by women who have migraine, but if the headaches get worse or cannot be controlled, or if other neurological symptoms occur, the pill should definitely be discontinued. It should also be noted that in addition to their other more deleterious and addictive effects, amphetamines and cocaine commonly cause headaches.

As discussed, even medications that are used to treat head pain can actually *cause* headaches. So if you start to experience chronic headaches, consider what medications you are currently taking. Daily use of prescription or over-the-counter medications designed to treat an acute headache may lead to chronic daily, or almost daily, headaches. The up-and-down fluctuations of the levels of these agents in the blood can result in daily rebound headaches. If this is the case, your physician should instruct you to gradually discontinue all pain medication for a certain period of time in order to separate the effects of the drug overuse from the original headache.

MEDICATIONS THAT MAY CAUSE REBOUND HEADACHES (CHRONIC TENSION HEADACHES) IF TAKEN DAILY

Over-the-Counter (OTC) Drugs
- acetaminophen (for example, Tylenol)
- aspirin and caffeine (for example, Anacin)
- acetaminophen, aspirin, and caffeine (e.g., Excedrin)

Prescription Drugs
- barbiturates in combinations with the above OTC products (for example, Esgic, Fiorinal)
- narcotics
  - propoxyphene (Darvon)
  - oxycodone with acetaminophen (Percocet or Tylox)

- hydrocodone bitartrate with acetaminophen (Vicodin)
- meperidine (Demerol)
- hydromorphone (Dilaudid)
- morphine

- ergotamine tartrate (for example, Cafergot)
- oral contraceptives
- heart medications
- medicines taken for other conditions

Chemicals

A large number of substances used in the workplace (including the artist's studio) can cause headaches in those people who work with them. These chemicals include various organic solvents, motor fuels, dyes, paints, and glues. Nitroglycerin, used in the production of dynamite, can cause headaches both by exposure and through withdrawal after habitual exposure (as when a worker in a munitions factory has time off from work). Carbon monoxide, from both automobiles and home-heating systems, can trigger headaches, as may air pollution from a variety of sources, including traffic, factories, and tobacco smoke in an enclosed room.

Miscellaneous External Triggers

Bright light. Sun in general, and particularly its glare off water, snow, or sand, may trigger headaches. The headache may involve a combination of muscle tension and vascular responses; squinting may bring on a tension headache, while the heat of the sun may help dilate blood vessels and trigger migraine. Wearing sunglasses is an important protective measure. Other bright lights, especially flickering lights, may also lead to headache.

Eyestrain. Eyestrain can cause an excessive contraction of the muscles in and around the eyes. This may occur when looking at a flickering computer screen for an extended time, for example, or scrutinizing the printed page in a closer and more detailed way than does the average reader. If your job entails close or detailed work, make sure you take a five-minute break at least once an hour. Gazing periodically around the room and changing the focus of your eyes from close to long range also can help prevent the muscles around the eyes from becoming strained.

Noise. High levels of unaccustomed noise can give anyone a headache. Examples abound—loud amplified music, noisy machinery, even yelling. Some of these headaches may be related to stress—when a teacher enters a noisy school lunchroom for the first time, for example, it might be the din, the stress of the situation, or the combination of both that triggers a headache. Similar types of stress may lead to the transient headache nearly all of us experience at one time or other. Over-the-counter medications usually help, although learning to relax and cope with the situation is a better way to prevent these headaches. Avoid loud noise since it can lead to eventual hearing loss. If you continue to get headaches from noise that you absolutely can't avoid (for example, machinery at work), then earplugs are the only answer.

Odors. Strong odors may trigger headaches. Migraine sufferers particularly may be sensitive to certain odors, and many report that their headaches are worse when they are exposed to certain aromas. The aromas, such as perfume or cooking odors, need not be unpleasant to evoke these reactions. Tobacco smoke is particularly difficult to tolerate when one has a headache.

Physical activity. A variety of physical factors may provoke or aggravate a headache. Even a slight bump on the head may bring on migraine. The English have coined the term *footballer's headache* for the headache that soccer players may get when they bounce the ball with their head. Headaches, particularly migraine, may be aggravated by such simple physical activity as climbing the stairs or bending over, or by sneezing or coughing. In certain predisposed individuals, the constant slight jarring that occurs when riding in a car may be enough to cause or worsen a headache.

Posture. Certain postures, particularly when they are held for a long time, can lead to muscle strain and headaches. If you sit much of the day with a telephone crooked between your neck and shoulder, bend over a typewriter or another piece of equipment for long periods of time, or perform any series of repetitive actions, you are vulnerable to experiencing muscle strain that can lead to a headache. Perhaps you unconsciously clench your jaw during the day or grind your teeth during sleep, habitually contracting your temporal muscles; these are all potential causes of headaches, and correcting such habits can help reduce their incidence. Wearing a cervical collar is sometimes helpful. If these measures fail, a physical therapist may offer useful advice or treatment.

Weather. Climatic changes, usually from good weather to bad, can trigger migraine and other types of headaches. (Some people can predict their migraines by changes in the weather and others can predict changes in the weather by the onset of their migraines.) Almost every type of weather has been implicated, but cloudy, gray days are the most common. Warm and humid weather is worse than cold, dry conditions, and the hot winds that prevail periodically in some countries are often blamed for triggering migraine.

Altitude. Ascending to high altitudes often causes headaches. The unacclimated person may get a headache (sometimes accompanied by nausea and vomiting) that is provoked by the vasodilation caused by the reduced oxygen content of the air. Amateur climbers should be aware that altitude sickness, a syndrome distinct from headache, is serious and can cause congestion of the lungs as well as the brain; death may result.

Internal Factors

Hormones. Hormonal factors in women are the most commonly implicated aggravating or precipitating internal components in migraine. As we have noted, migraine attacks often first begin at the time of puberty, approximately at the time that menstruation begins in young women. Migraine almost always disappears entirely during the mid- and last trimester of pregnancy, and it usually tapers off at menopause. Most commonly, migraine is triggered or aggravated around the time of menstruation. Despite these substantial hormonal implications, investigators have not found consistent hormonal changes in women with migraine when compared with those who have not had migraine.

It has been established that menstruation can often trigger migraine in women, and many women who don't normally experience migraine may also complain of headaches around the time of their menstrual periods. Migraine may be evoked by the sudden drop in estrodiol at menstruation. Other headaches may be related to fluid retention during menses. Menstrually related headaches often respond to treatment with over-the-counter pain relievers, but the nonsteroidal anti-inflammatory analgesics (for example, ibuprofen or naproxen) are particularly useful for menstrual migraine and headaches of the premenstrual syndrome.

Irregular body rhythms. Within our brains are "biological clocks" that regulate such periodic events as waking and sleeping, menstruation, and alterations in appetite. When these clocks are disturbed, such as occurs in jet lag, a headache may follow.

- *Sleeping.* In cluster headache patients, the individual attacks typically recur at the same time of the night during REM sleep, or they may occur during a daytime nap. Cluster periods also may recur at the same time every year. Migraine sufferers often awake in the morning with a headache. They often notice that their headaches are worse on weekends, which may be attributable to the fact that migraine occurs more frequently during periods of relaxation rather than stress. People also tend to sleep later on weekends than during the week. Paradoxically, sleeping too little as well as sleeping too much may bring on a migraine attack; irregularity in sleeping patterns may also provoke headaches.
- *Eating.* Missing a meal, going for extended periods without eating, or fasting often precipitates a headache. Researchers formerly believed that the headache resulted from a drop in blood sugar, as seen in diabetics who experience headaches when they are hypoglycemic. This concept, however, has not been confirmed. While some biochemical changes are certainly at work, the exact mechanism for headaches associated with fasting isn't known. Again, irregular eating habits can provoke a headache in susceptible people.

Emotional stress. Our internal reaction to emotional stress can be an important factor in provoking headaches. As noted, migraine typically does not occur during a period of stress, but usually upon relaxation *after* the initial stress is over. It's possible that residual anger and resentment may act as triggers, particularly if these emotions are chronically repressed. How we react to stress is an individual matter—what upsets some may have little or no effect on others. In addition, the reaction to stress varies greatly; some people respond emotionally (for example, rage) while others react physically (with a headache or upset stomach).

In any case, pain is a psychophysiological phenomenon. This means that a psychological reaction invariably accompanies the uncomfortable sensation. Normally, we cry when pain is severe. But chronic pain sufferers do not continuously cry; their psychological reaction to the pain is more subtle, and it may not even be apparent to the people who are experiencing the pain or to those around them. Unfortunately, this underlying psychological reaction may help to perpetuate the pain. Thus, psychological stress causes muscle tension, and excessive muscle tension causes pain. Chronic daily headaches or chronic tension headaches may be perpetuated by this vicious cycle.

If you suffer from chronic pain, you should be aware that a psychological reaction to the pain is normal. Accepting this fact will help you to cope with the pain and to learn particular pain-coping techniques that can help alleviate your condition (see chapter 5).

PSYCHOGENIC HEADACHES

We have seen that migraine and tension headaches can be triggered by various kinds of emotional stress. The emotions can play a role in triggering most types of headaches; cluster headache is the major exception.

In certain headaches, however, the emotions are the major, if not sole, cause of the headache. These are known as *psychogenic headaches*, and, contrary to popular opinion, are not common. Not only do they not involve physical or functional changes, but people with these headaches exhibit positive evidence of a psychological disturbance.

There are three main types of psychogenic headache: hysterical, depressive, and delusional.

The *conversion* or *hysterical* headache occurs when someone cannot cope with an emotional problem and subconsciously transforms it into a physical symptom, such as a headache. The pain, regardless of the process, is quite real.

Occasionally, headaches occur as physical manifestations of *depression*. Depression can disturb other body functions and cause insomnia, poor appetite, loss of sex drive—so, too, it may cause headache. Much more commonly, however, depression is a reaction to chronic pain. Depression lowers a person's pain threshold so that an irritant, normally only uncomfortable, may be felt as actual pain. Often it is impossible to determine whether the depression preceded or followed the sensation of chronic pain.

On rare occasions, the headache or other chronic pain is a *delusion*. The affected person has a false belief, contrary to obvious fact, that he or she is suffering severe or chronic pain. This is an indication of a serious psychological disturbance.

It must be kept in mind that psychogenic headaches are very real to those who suffer from them, and are as debilitating as other types of head pain. People with these headaches are often unable to function either at work or socially. The diagnosis and treatment is made only after a physician has ruled out any underlying disease or injury, as well as other nonorganic types of headaches.

People who experience psychogenic headaches usually have other psychological symptoms, so the diagnosis and treatment are best established in consultation with a psychologist or psychiatrist.

HEADACHES NAMED FOR THEIR TRIGGERS

Some rather unusual headaches are named after the factors that trigger them. Though they occur infrequently, they can be frightening to those who experience them, and deserve to be included here. These headaches are usually of short duration; people with migraine are particularly subject to them.

Headaches Caused by Sexual Activity

These headaches do not have to be associated with sexual intercourse—they can occur during masturbation, for example—nor do they need to be associated with orgasm. Furthermore, not all headaches associated with sexual activity are benign, for the exertion can cause the blowout of a cerebral aneurysm. Approximately 5 percent of all intracranial hemorrhages follow sexual activity.

The following case illustrates the difficulties in separating a headache due to a life-threatening hemorrhage from a benign headache associated with sexual intercourse.

John C., a 34-year-old married advertising executive, had an emergency consultation with one of the specialists at the headache unit. A few hours before, he had experienced "the worst headache in my life," and because he was familiar with medical literature, he was afraid that he had sustained a subarachnoid hemorrhage due to a ruptured aneurysm.

His physical and neurological examinations were normal, but the headache was in fact so typical of subarachnoid hemorrhage (see page 140) that a computerized tomogram (CAT scan) of the head was immediately ordered. The study was normal but not fully reassuring because a CAT scan is not capable of detecting a small amount of blood. Therefore, a spinal tap was recommended. The patient was reluctant to undergo this procedure because his pain had diminished. It was explained to him that severe headaches of short duration may be due to exertion, and he was asked again to review any activities that might have taken place just before the onset of the headache. He then sheepishly admitted that he had been having sexual intercourse with his secretary during lunch hour. This information, and the lessening of the pain, reassured the physician that the headache was probably due to sexual activity, although a small subarachnoid hemorrhage still was a possibility.

The physician made no comment on the nature of the situation, but asked to be notified if the headache should recur. The following day, the patient reported a recurrence of the headache under similar circumstances, and the physician then began to anticipate his patient's calls at one o'clock in the afternoon. After a series of severe headaches of short duration and without complications following intercourse, both the patient and his doctor were convinced that the headaches were associated with sexual activity and not due to hemorrhage. John C. eventually got a divorce and married his secretary. He reported that the sexually induced headaches disappeared after his remarriage and coincident with the decreased intensity of lovemaking.

Typically, the benign headache associated with sexual activity is a sudden, severe, throbbing pain over the back of the head or over the entire head. It usually lasts for only a few minutes, although sometimes the pain may persist for an hour or two. The condition occurs much more commonly in men than in women, and more often in people who suffer from migraine than in those who do not. It also occurs more often with sexual activity that is out of the ordinary, or "illicit." No doubt it was just this kind of headache to which Hippocrates was referring when he noted that a headache may be caused by "immoderate venery." The headache may occur before, during, or immediately after orgasm, and it is usually, but not necessarily, correlated with the degree of sexual excitement involved.

Several theories exist as to the mechanism of this sort of headache. Sexual activity causes an increase in muscle tension in all parts of the body; if a headache evolves gradually, it may take the form of a muscle contraction/muscle tension headache. More often, however, such a sexually induced headache has a sudden, throbbing migrainelike quality, probably because the increase in pulse, blood pressure, and blood vessel dilation associated with sexual activity evokes a similar mechanism.

The beta blocker propranolol (Inderal) is useful in preventing this type of headache, but this drug may also diminish potency or impair orgasm for both men and women. Other antimigraine medications or indomethacin may also be helpful. Periodic relaxation during sexual activity and recognition and avoidance of certain provoking positions or situations are also recommended.

Exertional and Cough Headache

Other types of physical exertion can bring on a headache. In particular, sudden *strenuous physical effort*, such as weight-lifting or moving a heavy object, may act as a trigger. Sometimes *coughing* may evoke a headache. It is believed that these headaches are the result of a brief increase in pressure within the head that occurs during exertion or other straining. When we exert ourselves strenuously or cough or sneeze, we perform an action called the *Valsalva maneuver*, in which we hold our breath and bear down. This causes a backing-up of blood and an associated increase in pressure within the head, presumably stretching blood vessels to cause pain.

This type of headache is usually sudden, sharp, and severe. It lasts only a minute or two, although, rarely, it may last considerably longer. Both sides of the head are affected. Men experience headache due to exertion more often than women, and those affected are usually between the ages of 30 and 70. Again, this sort of headache occurs more often in people who have migraine.

About half of those who experience exertional headache on a recurrent basis find that it stops after six months or so; even for others, the headaches eventually disappear. Indomethacin helps to prevent these attacks, and taking a medication containing ergotamine tartrate prior to exercise is also useful in preventing this troublesome pain. As with headache associated with sexual intercourse, a small percentage of patients with this presenting symptom are found to have a disease in the lower part or back of the head (cerebellum or brainstem). It follows, therefore, that if you experience these types of headaches, you should have a thorough neurological evaluation, including a computerized tomogram (CAT scan) or a magnetic resonance imaging (MRI) of the head.

Ice Cream Headache

When a cold substance is applied to the back of the mouth and the upper part of the throat, a sudden, severe headache may ensue. This pain is referred to as an *ice cream headache*, since the most common application of cold to these areas occurs when eating ice cream, especially in hot weather. The pain is sudden and severe, located behind the forehead or deep in the nose, but may also be in the temples or behind the cheeks. Fortunately, the headache lasts only 20 or 30 seconds, and disappears when the cold sensation abates.

It is thought that this kind of headache develops when the cold causes a reflex spasm of blood vessels in the mouth and throat, and that the associated deprivation of blood to the tissues causes the pain. Alternately, the vasospasm may cause a compensatory swelling of the blood vessels, briefly setting off a mechanism similar to that of migraine. Again, most patients with migraine will have experienced this type of headache at one time or another because they react to sudden changes in blood vessel tone much more readily than those who do not have migraine.

Swim-Goggle ("Tight-Hat") Headache

Sometimes a tight band around the head irritates the nerves of the scalp and causes headache. This often occurs with a hat that is too tight or, more commonly, with goggles worn to protect the eyes while swimming.

Other Headaches of Short Duration

In addition to the types of headaches triggered by various conditions and events, there are other headaches of short duration that do not have an obvious trigger. Their mechanisms are related to migraine and cluster headache. Most headaches of short duration usually respond well to indomethacin.

"Ice-pick headaches." These are severe, sharp, stabbing pains that are usually located within the temple or the back of the head. The pain may be a single jab or a series of jabs. Sometimes triggered by a sudden change in position or by exercise, they often occur without any provocation. The ice-pick headaches can also take place during a migraine attack or between attacks. Similarly, these stabbing pains may occur during a cluster headache, usually indicating the end of the attack.

Chronic paroxysmal hemicrania. This condition is one of the forms of cluster headache described earlier. Located in and around one eye, it usually lasts for only a few minutes, but it recurs many times a day. Unlike other forms of cluster headache, chronic paroxysmal hemicrania occurs more commonly in women than in men. This type of headache can always be prevented by indomethacin.

Hemicrania continua. A rare type of headache, this is a chronic, continuous, one-sided pain that goes on for months or years. It is mentioned here, even though it is not of short duration, because it, too, is responsive to indomethacin.

It's important to remember that most types of headache can be alleviated. If you think your headaches are related to a specific trigger, be sure to make a point of telling it to your physician. Armed with your examination results, your medical history, and your description of symptoms, the doctor can then make the correct diagnosis and recommend the appropriate treatment.

5

Nondrug Therapies

Physicians are sometimes justly criticized for not considering the patient as a whole. In the treatment of headache patients, this attitude might involve a preoccupation with the headache itself as a localized pain without regard to the patient's complete medical history, home life, work, social environment, and personality. Holistic medicine is not a recent development; considering every aspect of a patient's life, whether or not these aspects immediately appear to be related to the primary symptom, has been the basis of sound medical practice for the last century. As we have seen, most headaches, particularly recurring headaches, are not simply a matter of a "pain in the head."

The physician's proper role is to diagnose and treat your headaches *and* attempt to enhance your overall quality of life. While it's true that many doctors don't practice from such a broad perspective, it's also true that many patients come to a doctor for a "quick fix"—they want an immediate remedy for their headaches so that they can get on with their lives. Thus there is an inclination on the part of both physicians and patients to depend on available drugs as a palliative. As we have seen when examining migraine and tension headaches, however, the overuse of either prescription or over-the-counter medications can lead to the rebound and severe exacerbation of head pain. In fact, *all* the medications used to treat headaches, whether prescription or over-the-counter, are associated with potential side effects. It is just as important to remember that no medication can guarantee complete relief from headaches. Despite the proclivity of both patient and doctor to look to medication as the major treatment for recurrent headaches, a number of nondrug therapies are available that can offer substantial and lasting relief for the headache patient. These therapies include:

- Eliminating or reducing the factors that appear to trigger or aggravate the headaches.
- Practicing various relaxation techniques and taking other physical measures that can help relieve or prevent headaches.
- Paying attention to psychological factors.

We have surveyed some of these nondrug procedures in previous chapters; here we place them in perspective as practical strategies.

ELIMINATING TRIGGERING AND AGGRAVATING FACTORS

As noted before, there's a long list of factors that can either trigger or exacerbate various types of headaches, including alcohol and a variety of foods in the case of migraine; emotional stress and daily intake of analgesics in the case of tension headaches; and alcohol in the case of cluster headaches. It is important to realize that reducing or eliminating such triggering factors can greatly reduce the frequency and/or severity of your headaches (see chapter 4 and diet recommendations for patients with migraine).

Factors other than food also are known to trigger, aggravate, or perpetuate headaches. Finding alternatives for certain medications used for heart disease and birth control, for example, may eliminate your head pain. Gradually discontinuing the always inadvisable daily use of medicine designed for occasional treatment of headache and other pain may entirely relieve chronic daily headaches. Restoring the regularity of sleeping, eating, or other disturbances in life-style is another method of abolishing or diminishing a variety of headaches.

Giving up favorite foods or beverages, or ensuring regular eating and sleeping patterns may be trying, but eliminating stress from your life is a far more difficult task, if not an impossible one. Stress is, after all, part of the human condition. Learning to cope with the various stresses of daily life, and thus reducing their impact, is certainly more practical than trying to isolate yourself from stress.

RELAXATION TECHNIQUES

Relaxation can play an important role in helping to reduce the frequency or severity of your migraine and tension headaches. True relaxation isn't easy; even when we aren't undergoing immediate emotional stress, our minds and muscles stay active. Because attempting to relax is often more difficult than assumed, it is usually wise to have the help of personal instruction and special techniques to achieve the benefits of complete relaxation.

What has been termed *deep relaxation* or the *relaxation response* involves altering body function to promote a sense of detachment and well-being. This includes relaxing muscles in the head, neck, and the rest of the body. When deep relaxation is achieved there is a marked decrease in muscle tension; heart and respiratory rate may also decrease.

You may find that simply lying down and closing your eyes during a headache provides some relief. As we know, migraine sufferers instinctively tend to lie down in a dark, quiet room. Other people suffering from headaches try to relax by getting away and taking a walk. Massaging the neck and head muscles can help relieve the pain, as can applying cold compresses to the head, which theoretically diminishes the swelling of the blood vessels. Paradoxically, applying warm compresses may also help, probably by enhancing muscle relaxation. But if you suffer from recurrent headaches, you've probably tried these measures yourself and found that they provide only partial relief, without producing a sense of deep relaxation.

Deep relaxation is a technique that can be learned, with practice. What's more, relaxation can be used in two different ways as a treatment for headaches: the first is employed to diminish or curtail the pain while the headache is in progress; the second involves practicing relaxation on a regular basis every day or at least several times a week to help prevent headaches.

Most people understand intuitively that there is a relationship between muscular tension, emotional stress, and headaches, but they aren't able to do anything about it on their own. That's why learning relaxation exercises under the supervision of a specialist in the field is highly recommended. Relaxation therapy works best when it is structured.

Probably the simplest form of relaxation exercise is progressive relaxation, which consists of lying down and concentrating on different parts of your body, one at a time. As you alternately contract and release specific muscles in a set pattern, you become aware of how much unnecessary tension is sustained by these muscles much of the time. In one progressive relaxation exercise, you start with your legs, contracting the muscles for 20 seconds, and then slowly "let go." You do the same with your back, abdomen, arms, neck, forehead, eyes, and jaw. Once you *genuinely* relax each part of your body, you'll find that you're able to lie still quite calmly for five minutes or more, letting your mind drift in a serene and pleasant fashion. Here is one possible format for progressive relaxation; note that different instructors may follow slightly different procedures.

Progressive Relaxation Techniques

1. Lie down. Close your eyes.
2. Concentrate on the muscles in your lower legs; first contract them for 20 seconds; feel the tightness in the muscles, and then let go and relax them, slowly and steadily. Rest in the relaxed state for 20 to 30 seconds.
3. Perform the same procedure with your other muscle groups, one at a time, slowly moving up along your body: thighs, buttocks, abdomen, chest, shoulders, neck, jaw, forehead.
4. Lie still for several minutes, letting your thoughts float.

Most people can only half-relax when they first start out, so having a professional supervise you, at least the first few times, is worthwhile. In this way you will know if you are performing the exercise correctly and learn the amount of time you should spend on each muscle group. At first, the idea may seem odd, but the supervisor will make sure that you're doing the right procedure, so you can use the technique on your own later. This is not a quick fix. It's also important to remember that you shouldn't push yourself or try too hard to relax; instead, maintain a passive attitude, allowing the body to relax itself. Eventually, the relaxation response becomes natural and you can incorporate it into your daily regimen without first going through the muscle-contraction phase.

Other relaxation exercises that don't involve special equipment include relaxing by listening to relaxation tapes, doing deep-breathing exercises, or practicing the techniques of transcendental meditation, autosuggestion, or yoga. Hypnosis training has also been used successfully in some headache patients to help elicit the relaxation response.

Biofeedback Techniques

Biofeedback is a means of monitoring and controlling otherwise unconscious or involuntary physical processes through the use of special equipment. The techniques benefit the patient and relieve the headache by evoking a generalized relaxation response that affects the body as a whole. In addition, and perhaps more important, learning to control such bodily functions as skin temperature and muscle tone give patients a sense of self-control. If they can control these involuntary activities of the body, they feel they can probably control and relieve their headaches.

How can you be certain that muscles of the head and neck are relaxed? If you're told to relax your arm, you can see and feel it drop to your side, but you can't see or feel your scalp muscles relax. That's where biofeedback is effective, because it allows you to monitor those body responses that are not under your obvious conscious control. If you can learn to voluntarily produce specific changes in your body—a decrease in scalp muscle tension, for example—you are on the way to establishing a degree of control over at least some of the physical changes that may lead to a headache.

During biofeedback training, people are taught relaxation techniques, such as imagining a calm situation, and are given the choice of using the one that works best. By means of the biofeedback equipment, they can then observe how successful they are at relaxing specific muscles. Most people can learn to achieve an adequate and measurable degree of relaxation after 10 or fewer biofeedback training sessions. The relaxation techniques learned at the biofeedback clinic are practiced daily at home to ensure maximum effectiveness. As with many beneficial techniques, motivation is a prime prerequisite.

The most common biofeedback procedure uses electromyography (EMG). Electrodes, pasted on the forehead or face, transmit electrical impulses, generated by the contraction of the underlying muscles. The degree of muscle tension is translated into a series of sounds (clicks, beeps) or visual images (blinking lights or movements of a hand on a dial). The faster this electronic response, the more tense the muscles. Conversely, learning to slow the response—that is, slowing the clicks or lights—is correlated with the degree of relaxation. Once you learn the techniques that produce muscle relaxation, you must continue to practice them on your own. Studies have shown that headache sufferers can learn to reduce the intensity of their muscle tension by as much as 50 percent to 70 percent by biofeedback.

Another common type of biofeedback training is temperature regulation of the skin. A small device that can pick up slight changes in the temperature of the skin is attached to one of your fingers, and you are taught how to raise the temperature. Again, you can see or hear how successful you are by way of the biofeedback equipment. Changing skin temperature is an indirect way of altering blood flow to the skin. One theory maintains that an increase in blood flow to the hand, with dilation of these blood vessels, causes compensatory constriction of the blood vessels in the scalp, and thus a beneficial effect on migraine, but this mechanism has never been proved. Nevertheless, inducing hand-warming produces a general relaxation response.

Biofeedback, like other forms of relaxation training, requires practice. It has been shown that *daily* rather than occasional use of biofeedback or other relaxation techniques confers the greatest benefit, particularly as far as preventing headaches. Biofeedback is also employed successfully by migraine patients to abort or diminish individual attacks. Like medications used for similar purposes, biofeedback, if practiced at the very onset of migraine, can often curtail the attack. If you are to succeed with this technique, you must first learn how to invoke a relaxation response and then be able to use it at will—at work, at play, or at home.

As we noted earlier, most people need structured training if substantial benefit is to be derived from relaxation exercises, and such training is essential for the proper use of biofeedback techniques. Courses in biofeedback or other relaxation techniques, whether arranged through a physician, a psychologist, or a relaxation specialist, may be expensive and time-consuming. However, it's often more than offset by savings in the amount of headache medication otherwise consumed. You may still require medication for some acute headaches, but relaxation can help reduce your reliance on drugs and will often diminish both the frequency and the severity of your pain.

SPECIAL PAIN-RELIEF TECHNIQUES

Some of the other methods of altering body function as a way of diminishing pain are used infrequently in the treatment of headaches, partly because they are impractical. *Transcutaneous electrical nerve stimulation (TENS)* is a treatment by which a series of tiny, painless electrical shocks are delivered to the skin overlying a painful area. This technique can reduce pain, but it is not in common use for treating headaches, largely because of the cumbersome nature of the equipment. *Acupuncture* and *acupressure,* based on needle puncturing or pressure to specific areas of the skin, are ancient Chinese methods for relieving pain, and they are used with some success today in a variety of circumstances. Again, however, it is impractical to run to an acupuncturist whenever you get a headache, and, unfortunately, TENS and acupuncture do nothing to *prevent* headaches.

The mechanisms by which TENS and acupuncture or acupressure relieve pain are not known. They may alter the pain impulse by shutting off certain relay centers in the nervous system (pain gates), or by stimulating production of the body's own natural pain relievers (the endorphins and enkephalins), or by a combination of these actions.

Hypnosis also may help a bout of headache, and some people can be taught, in a sense, to hypnotize themselves during a headache so as not to feel the pain.

Sometimes, muscles tighten into knots and cause pain. When pressure on these areas elicits headache pain, they are known as *trigger points*. Injecting these points with a *local anesthetic* or simply inserting a needle into them may block the pain mechanism. Certain nerves of the head, particularly the occipital nerve that supplies sensation to the back of the scalp, may be compressed by muscles or by scar tissue. Similarly, the nerve roots from the neck that lead to the occipital nerve may become pinched by the excessive growth of bone caused by conditions like arthritis. Such irritation of the nerve or nerve roots causes pain, which may be experienced as a headache. This kind of pain can be relieved by blocking the nerve with local anesthetics, a technique that has been used successfully for pain relief in severe cases of cluster headache (see chapter 3) and for occipital neuralgia (see page 150). It may also interfere with the pain mechanisms of other headaches.

Other Physical Measures

Certain other first-aid techniques can temporarily alter the physiology of the body and relieve headache pain. As we noted earlier, many patients use *cold or hot compresses.* Cold constricts the blood vessels and may thus decrease the dilation that is an important part of the pain mechanism involved in migraine; heat helps to relax the muscles and relieves the pain of tension headache. *Rubbing the area that hurts* is no doubt an instinctive response to pain. Indeed, rubbing the temples may relieve migraine, and massage of painful or tender scalp, neck, or shoulder muscles may help with bouts of tension headache or migraine. Patients with migraine find that compressing the blood vessels at the temple diminishes the throbbing pain. However, the pain comes back when the pressure is released, so many migraine sufferers tie a tight band around their head. Regular aerobic exercise also is thought to be helpful for some patients.

The administration of 100 percent oxygen constricts blood vessels and is useful in aborting acute cluster headache attacks; it requires medical supervision and access to an oxygen tank or canister and mask (see chapter 3). *Carbon dioxide* is a powerful dilator of blood vessels and is sometimes used to abort the aura of migraine. The sufferer simply breathes in and out inside a paper bag. This must, however, be done during the aura: once the headache phase has started, the carbon dioxide may make the attack worse.

PSYCHOLOGICAL MANAGEMENT

Many headache patients are reluctant to acknowledge the relationship between headache and emotional or psychological factors. Comments such as "I'm not crazy," or "The pain is *real!*" are common. While such statements are true, anyone who experiences recurrent headaches must recognize that pain (particularly chronic pain) *always* entails a psychological component, and acknowledging this casts no aspersions on the state of one's mental health. If pain is severe enough, we will cry. Less severe pain may not evoke the same reaction, but it nevertheless initiates an emotional response, one that patients don't necessarily reveal to friends, family, co-workers, or, sometimes, even to themselves. Realizing that emotional factors are a normal component of pain is an important first step toward relieving that pain.

Headaches are not necessarily directly caused by emotional stress, although stress can trigger them. Tension headaches tend to increase as emotional stress builds up. Migraine attacks, on the other hand, most commonly occur after a stressful incident is over, hence their frequent occurrence on weekends and during vacations. The emotional disturbance need not be severe, and its precise role in initiating or exacerbating headaches is related to the underlying personality of the sufferer. We all react differently to stress. Some people seem to cope easily with it. Some of us don't and develop a peptic ulcer, while others develop high blood pressure. In yet other people, the stress does not seem to cause any apparent physical reaction, but it may act in other, less obvious ways. In susceptible individuals, the predictable stresses of everyday life, combined with the other components that trigger headaches, are often sufficient to initiate a headache.

Because emotional reactions are an integral response to the experience of pain, it is not surprising that people with chronic pain develop behavioral and psychological reactions. These, in turn, may perpetuate or aggravate the pain. Behavioral reactions are often manifested by sleep disturbances with associated fatigue and irritability. Diminished physical activity is usually first manifested by withdrawal from social interactions. Overuse of medication is part of the behavioral changes of chronic headache sufferers. Some of these changes may be the first manifestation of psychological reactions, especially depression or anxiety or both.

If you feel that your headaches are a reflection of your personality, some kind of proof that you can't handle stressful situations that other people seem to manage quite well, you should understand that the headaches are not necessarily related to a *specific* stressful event. They may simply be your body's reaction to the many accumulated stresses of everyday life.

The psychological reaction to pain can take many forms, and the most common are depression and anxiety. The depression may not be obvious; many depressed people may simply have difficulty sleeping, or report a loss of appetite, or, less often, may eat excessively. The particularly unfortunate factor about such a response is that psychological reactions such as depression and anxiety lower the threshold of pain and can make the painful condition worse, thus setting up a vicious cycle of pain, depression, anxiety, and more pain. On occasion, the headache itself may be the sole manifestation of depression.

Most patients with chronic pain do not wince or cry, so the people around them may not appreciate the severity of their pain. Family members, co-workers, and friends may not understand how disabling headaches can be, since they have no real way of gauging the sufferer's degree of pain or discomfort. As a result, patients' associates may be unsympathetic, or may even accuse them of exaggerating or faking their pain. This reaction is a major source of repressed anger in the chronic headache sufferer.

It is extremely important that physicians listen carefully to what their headache patients tell them. A physician doesn't need to be Sigmund Freud to allow the patient to ventilate repressed anger or to discuss the aspects of life that may cause stress or may involve other serious psychological burdens. People often repress memories of childhood abuse or the existence of chronic problems in the workplace or in relations with family or friends. The doctor may be able to offer valuable counseling with regard to these problems in interpersonal relationships.

Worrying that your headaches are due to a brain tumor or another serious underlying disease is certainly understandable. Your medical history and thorough physical and neurological examinations usually allow a physician to rule out any serious organic condition. If there is any doubt at all, the doctor will order further tests, such as a computerized X-ray tomogram of the head (CAT scan) or magnetic resonance imaging (MRI). Occasionally, reassurance alone is enough to diminish a patient's anxiety, and thus diminish the frequency and severity of headaches.

Some patients may have emotional problems that are not readily solved: a woman who has a husband who is emotionally or physically abusive and children who are unmanageable, for example. However, even in such cases, stress reduction is possible. A change of environment may help; sometimes just getting out of the house and taking a walk can do wonders. A longer period of change, such as a vacation, also may be strongly recommended.

The Role of a Psychiatrist or Psychologist in Headache Relief

Only rarely are a headache sufferer's psychological problems so severe that they require psychotherapy with a psychologist or psychiatrist. More often, these professionals are consulted to teach headache patients specific behavioral or mental techniques for coping with pain, so that they can learn to ameliorate the headaches on their own. This is accomplished partly by learning to recognize some of the situations that trigger or aggravate the headache, and then to avoid or diminish these particular events or stresses. In other cases, the mental health professionals consulted may find subconsciously hidden reasons for depression, anxiety, anger, guilt, and other factors that may be outwardly experienced as headaches, and on these occasions psychotherapy may constitute an integral part of headache treatment.

Cognitive-behavioral therapy. Headache management involves the education and training of patients in pain-coping techniques; these may be termed *cognitive-behavioral therapy* (also called *pain-coping* and *stress-coping therapy*). All physicians engage in such therapy, although it may not be labeled as such. When doctors advise patients to change their eating or drinking habits, ask them to maintain regular patterns of sleep, or avoid daily pain medication (to name a few examples), they are engaging in behavioral therapy. More formal behavioral management teaches the patient new behaviors and new skills to blunt rather than enhance pain mechanisms. Relaxation exercises are an example. Patients are taught how to tolerate and participate in activities formerly shunned. Attempts are made to modify certain personality traits such as those found in the hard-driving, aggressive, Type-A personality.

The cognitive aspects of therapy attempt to change the thinking patterns of chronic headache sufferers. First, patients must recognize the relationship between emotions and pain (headache). Then they must identify those reactions that may trigger or aggravate a headache. Finally, patients are taught to develop alternate reactions or thoughts to help fend off those factors that bring on the headache.

The mental imaging that people use in biofeedback treatment to evoke relaxation can be considered an example of cognitive therapy. However, psychologists and psychiatrists use a much wider range of techniques. Patients may learn certain interpersonal skills—for example, assertiveness. They may learn how to communicate their problems to others without evoking pity or guilt and how to ventilate anger without irritating loved ones or friends.

Specific cognitive pain-coping techniques involve the modification of thought processes. Patients may learn how to divert their attention away from the pain, by repeating in one's mind pleasant thoughts, by praying, by engaging in mental tasks, or by changing activities. Patients are taught not to engage in negative thinking. They are instructed not to anticipate that the headache will get worse, but rather tell themselves "I've had the headache before, I've come through it well, it's not so bad."

None of these nondrug therapies, including the elimination or reduction of triggering factors, offers a magic fix for the "cure" of your headaches. But in combination with each other or with the proper use of medication, they can significantly reduce the impact headaches have on your life.

6

Controversial Headaches

As many as 40 million people in the United States experience some form of recurrent headaches. With such widespread incidence, it isn't surprising that many headache sufferers have misconceptions about the cause of their headaches. Sometimes these misconceptions are the result of popular magazine articles or advertising campaigns on behalf of the manufacturers of headache remedies. Sometimes the cause of the headache is misdiagnosed by a physician or dentist. But in still other cases, the nature of the headache is a matter of controversy among medical authorities themselves. What follows surveys some of the most common of these controversial, problematic headaches.

SINUS AND ALLERGIC HEADACHES

Many people believe that they suffer from what they refer to as "sinus" headaches. Nearly everyone is familiar with the dramatic illustrations of "sinus headache" that have appeared on television, with arrows pointing to the alleged site of the pain. As one result of such campaigns, many people regard headaches that are associated with the clogging of the nasal passages as being attributable to their sinuses. For the great majority of patients, this simply isn't the case.

Certainly acute infection of the paranasal sinuses (around the nose) will cause pain in the overlying areas of the face and head. When acute infection of the sinuses is present (*acute sinusitis*), there is swelling and tenderness over the sinus area, fever, and a generalized feeling of sickness. In such infections, the fever and illness that affect the body as a whole may be more troublesome than the head or face pain.

Most people who believe they suffer from sinus headaches attribute them to *chronic sinusitis* or to an "allergy." It is true that a blocked sinus, a cyst within the sinus, or chronic sinus inflammation may sometimes cause headaches, but headaches due to these conditions are relatively rare.

Low-grade sinusitis, allergic reaction of the upper respiratory tract, and headache are common. These conditions often occur together by coincidence. Just because a headache occurs when you are experiencing a clogged or draining nose does not mean that the headache has an allergic basis. Similarly, if allergy testing reveals a sensitivity to dust, pollen, or other allergens, it doesn't mean that your headaches are "allergic." Indeed, headaches rarely have an allergic basis.

Most patients who think their headaches are caused by chronic or allergic sinusitis are eventually found to have either migraine or tension headaches, both of which are far more common than headaches due to sinus disease or an allergy.

As we have seen, patients with cluster headache are sometimes misdiagnosed as having either sinusitis or an allergic reaction (see chapter 3). The redness and tearing of the eye, as well as the clogging of and the discharge from the nose, lead the patient and sometimes the examining physician to conclude that the headaches are due to local changes in the membranes of the nose, sinuses, and eyes. Physicians who obtain a detailed history from the patient are usually able to differentiate cluster headaches from acute or chronic sinusitis.

If you or your physician believe you may be suffering from what is all too often termed "sinus headache," make certain that you describe *all* your symptoms carefully to the physician, including when and under what circumstances the headaches occur. X-ray examination is often employed to determine whether sinus abnormalities are present. But a minor change seen in the X-ray films, such as thickening of the sinus lining or evidence of a low-grade inflammation, does not mean the headaches are due to sinus disease. While the possibility of sinus problems should not be automatically dismissed, the chances are that your headaches have another cause.

TEMPOROMANDIBULAR JOINT (TMJ) DYSFUNCTION SYNDROME

The temporomandibular joint (TMJ) acts as a hinge between the upper and lower jaws and lies just in front of each ear. When the TMJ is the site of arthritis, infection, or other injury, then pain, sometimes quite intense, occurs in and around the joint and may extend beyond it into the face, temple, or other parts of the head. However, the *TMJ dysfunction syndrome* refers to what is presumed to be a disturbance in the function of this joint and not to obvious disease; whether the pain in the area of the TMJ is actually due to altered function of the joint or should be attributed to spasm of the muscles that open and close the jaw is currently a matter of controversy. The term *myofascial pain dysfunction (MPD)* is used when the muscles involved in chewing appear to be involved.

There are three major features of TMJ disease or the TMJ

131

dysfunction syndrome. First, the pain is aggravated by using the jaw, particularly when chewing hard food. Second, because of the pain (jaw dysfunction or muscle spasm) the patient's ability to open the jaw fully is impaired. Third, there is tenderness in the area of the joint and/or its muscles. A click or other sound heard when the jaw is opened and closed is sometimes related to TMJ dysfunction, but such clicks are extremely common in the general population and are not usually important.

The International Headache Society favors the concept of spasm in the muscle rather than a disturbance in the joint as an explanation for the condition termed TMJ dysfunction syndrome. The symptoms of TMJ dysfunction would thus be attributed to the same factors that cause tension headache. The muscles of the scalp are chiefly involved in tension headaches; the muscles of the face, including the chewing muscles, are involved in the facial pain attributed to TMJ disorder.

Regardless of the exact mechanism involved, no more than conservative treatment for TMJ dysfunction or myofascial pain dysfunction is recommended, The patient should rest the jaw and avoid chewing hard foods. Locally applied heat may be helpful. If nighttime jaw clenching is present, it can be diminished with a bite plate. Medication, if required, is similar to that used for tension headaches: over-the-counter analgesics or prescription medications, especially nonsteroidal anti-inflammatory pain relievers (for example, naproxen), and centrally acting analgesics such as the tricyclic antidepressants (for example, amitriptyline hydrochloride). (See chapter 2, where these medications, including their proper use and most common side effects, are described in detail.) Surgery for TMJ dysfunction should be avoided.

HEADACHES AFTER HEAD INJURY

Post-traumatic or *postconcussion headaches* can be devastating, even when very little if any objective evidence of disease or residual brain injury is found. These headaches most often appear after a closed head injury—that is, a head injury not associated with skull fracture. The head injury is usually not severe enough to cause a contusion (bruise) or laceration of the brain. When these severe injuries to the brain do occur, there are obvious neurological signs, such as weakness on one side of the body or impairment of vision. People who have sustained mild head injuries may briefly lose consciousness (a concussion), but headaches may follow without even this symptom.

People whose headaches persist long after mild head injuries often experience a number of other symptoms that do not reveal any associated physical changes when examined. In addition to headaches, they may complain of dizziness, memory impairment, difficulty in concentrating, decreased attention span, and decreased sexual desire. More troubling, the person often undergoes a noticeable change in emotional character, with the development of depression or sudden bursts of anger, often seemingly without cause. These symptoms may be sufficiently disabling to prevent the person from working effectively. Nevertheless, the results of standard physical and neurological examinations are usually normal, as are the CAT scans or MRIs of the head and most other neurological tests.

What causes this condition is still a matter of conjecture. It is known that even a mild head injury can cause the brain to be shaken or swirled within the confines of the skull. This disturbance may lead to subtle changes in the brain that may be evident only with the most powerful electron microscopes.

Chronic post-traumatic headache occurs more often after mild head injuries than after severe injuries that cause obvious damage to the brain. Fracturing of the skull absorbs a great deal of energy, and in so doing protects the brain, just as cracking an egg will leave the yolk intact. On the other hand, severe acceleration and deceleration of the head, as in a whiplash injury, will not fracture the skull but may shake up the brain in such a way as to cause headache, dizziness, and other symptoms, just as shaking an egg may rupture the yolk without cracking the shell.

In the past, post-traumatic headaches that were not associated with any observable physical changes were often considered to be psychogenic in nature, related more to the psychological rather than the physical trauma of an accident or to the medical-legal issues that are often involved. This is no longer considered to be the case, except in a small minority of patients. In cases where litigation is pending (as with a motor vehicle accident), patients may be accused of fabricating their headaches as a strategy to win a larger amount in damages. It should be noted, however, that legal settlements favorable to these patients usually do not resolve their symptoms. Although objective physical evidence of residual head injury is lacking and headache and other symptoms are difficult or impossible to document, some neurological-functional tests are useful. Psychometric evaluations of mental capacity and other sophisticated studies, may help to determine impairment in a patient's capability even when physical evidence is absent.

The characteristics of the post-traumatic headache usually resemble those of tension headache or, less often, migraine; the treatment is basically the same as for these headaches. Nonpharmacologic therapy may be helpful and vocational rehabilitation may be needed. Physicians should provide patients with sympathy and understanding; patients whose physicians are unable to do so should consult another practitioner in the field. It is also vital that family, friends, and employers be assured that the symptoms are real and not psychological in nature, so that they may offer the patient emotional support. Most of these headaches gradually clear up within six months to two years, but in some people the symptoms are more or less permanent.

HIGH BLOOD PRESSURE AND HEADACHES

Many patients tell their physicians that they know when their blood pressure is high because that's when they have a headache. Yet high blood pressure and headache rarely have a direct relationship with one another. Since hypertension and headaches are both common conditions, their occurrence at the same time is usually purely coincidental. Essential hypertension—that is, hypertension that isn't secondary to some other factor—is the most common form of high blood pressure and, contrary to popular opinion, does not *in itself* cause headaches. Only in rare instances, when blood pressure rises precipitously to very high levels—a reading of 270/130, for example—does headache occur.

Such sudden rises in blood pressure are associated with certain tumors of the adrenal gland, which are related to the excessive secretion of adrenaline; with the transformation of benign to severe or "malignant" hypertension; or with toxemia of pregnancy (*eclampsia*). Such sudden and severe rises in blood pressure can cause a swelling of the brain, headache, and may lead to stroke.

LOW BLOOD SUGAR AND HEADACHE

Another condition that is falsely assumed to be a common cause of headaches is hypoglycemia. For most of us, the level of sugar in the blood normally fluctuates during the day, rising after a meal and falling three to four hours later. Most patients who have been told that they are hypoglycemic have what is termed *functional hypoglycemia*, which means only that their blood sugar sometimes drops below the standard normal range. Usually, this functional hypoglycemia is falsely blamed for symptoms that either cannot be explained readily or are psychological in origin. True hypoglycemia, on the other hand, most commonly occurs in people who are diabetic and take an excessive amount of insulin; in diabetics, true hypoglycemia will cause headaches as well as many other symptoms, including weakness, palpitations, and tremors. The point here is that functional hypoglycemia in an otherwise normal individual is not usually associated with headaches.

HEADACHE AND THE NECK

There is a great deal of medical controversy regarding the role of the neck area as a cause of headache. Interestingly, the diagnosis of *cervicogenic headache*—headache originating in the bones, ligaments, or muscles of the neck—is made far more often by European physicians than by their American counterparts. Many people who have severe arthritis of the neck experience little or no pain, although there is no doubt that arthritis or a herniated disk may pinch a nerve root, causing considerable pain in the neck and shoulder; the pain may then radiate up into the head.

Whiplash injuries often cause pain in the head and neck that gradually disappears as the stretched or torn muscles and ligaments heal. More severe whiplash injuries can fracture vertebrae or cause herniated disks. A neurological examination and X-rays of the neck can establish the cause of the pain. Wearing a cervical collar affords relief for most patients with this condition. Chiropractic manipulation of the lower back to relieve local pain in that area may be helpful for some, but manipulation of the neck to relieve headache rarely makes scientific sense and may be dangerous.

7

Headaches Due
to Disease

While 90 percent of headaches fit into one of the three functional or nonorganic headache classifications (migraine, tension headache, or cluster headache), literally hundreds of causes exist for the remaining 10 percent, namely, those which are associated with an underlying disease. These organic headaches are attributable either to disease located within the head or to disease that affects the body as a whole, as well as to head and face pains caused by local disease or by disorders of the cranial nerves. How these conditions cause headaches is described here.

DISEASES IN THE HEAD

Diseases Causing Changes of Pressure in the Head

The brain is insensitive to pain; thus, many of the disorders that affect it will not cause a headache until the disease itself spreads and takes up more space than is available in the confined skull cavity. The diseases that take up space include *tumors, abscesses,* and *blood clots* (*hematomas*). All these conditions will cause headaches, either by stretching the coverings of the brain (the *meninges*) or by stretching the pain-sensitive blood vessels that are located predominantly at the base of the brain.

Many people fear that they have a brain tumor when their headaches first appear. Fortunately, the headache associated with a brain tumor (or abscess or hematoma) possesses certain characteristics that help to distinguish it from nonorganic headaches such as migraine, tension headaches, or cluster headaches. Specifically, a brain tumor usually causes a headache that is recognized as being of relatively recent origin, as opposed to one that has been recurring over time. The headache is usually one-sided, and located approximately over the tumor; if the tumor is at the base of the brain, the headache is usually located at the back of the head. Headaches associated with brain tumor are often worse in the morning and exacerbated by head movement, but these features are also true of migraine. *Most distinctive, the head pain associated with a brain tumor tends to increase in severity, duration, and frequency until it becomes continuous.*

The diagnosis of brain tumor, however, is not usually made on the basis of headache characteristics, but rather by determining the presence of associated symptoms and certain signs that are referable to the brain. Generalized disturbances may be evident, such as changes in personality, impairment of memory or other intellectual functions, drowsiness, or convulsions. Localized disturbances of brain function may also be apparent, such as weakness or numbness of one part of the body or vision disturbances. *When these or other neurological symptoms accompany headache, a physician's attention is mandatory and a CAT scan or MRI of the head is advisable.*

Organic headaches also can be caused by an increase in the size of the brain, produced by tissue swelling or by the enlargement of the brain's cavities (ventricles). This swelling of the brain can occur as a result of a number of conditions, most notably, *encephalitis* (inflammation of the brain). Encephalitis causes fever and a generalized disturbance of brain function, including drowsiness and mental confusion.

Whatever the cause of the excessive pressure within the head, examination may reveal swelling of the optic nerves (papilledema). Headaches with papilledema are often caused by a brain tumor, but if no other symptoms or signs are present, they may also be caused by brain *edema* (fluid retention in the brain) and are then termed *pseudotumor cerebri* of the brain. For unknown reasons, young obese women who have menstrual difficulties are particularly subject to this condition. The excessive use of vitamin A and certain antibiotics, as well as other factors, may also lead to brain swelling with headache and papilledema. *Hydrocephalus* (swelling of the cavities of the brain) occurs when the outflow of cerebrospinal fluid from the cavities of the brain is blocked or poorly absorbed. It is characterized by difficulties in walking, impairment of intellectual function, and urinary incontinence, with or without generalized headache.

After a spinal tap, cerebrospinal fluid may leak into the tissues of the back through the puncture wound. The loss of this fluid causes unusually low pressure (or negative pressure) within the head whenever the patient sits up or stands; this low pressure stretches the meninges and the basal blood vessels, producing severe headache. The headache disappears when the patient lies down, only to return when he or she sits up or stands again. It may take several days for the puncture wound to heal. As the cerebrospinal fluid is replenished, the pressure returns to normal and the headache disappears. If the headache persists for more than a few days, the physician may seal the puncture wound with a blood patch: a small amount of the patient's blood is injected into the area of the former puncture; the blood clots and seals both the old and new punctures.

Irritation of the Meninges

The most common cause of meningeal irritation is blood. The subarachnoid space between the brain and the skull is occupied by the cerebrospinal fluid that acts as a shock absorber. When blood enters this space, it increases intracranial pressure and results in a headache. In addition, the blood itself has an irritating effect on the meninges and causes a stiff neck as well as a severe headache. When an aneurysm (the ballooning of a weakened blood vessel) or a tangle of blood vessels (arteriovenous malformation) ruptures within the head, it causes *subarachnoid hemorrhage*.

The sudden onset of very severe headache is the distinguishing characteristic of subarachnoid hemorrhage, which is often fatal. In fact, *any* headache that begins suddenly and is unusually severe may be due to a subarachnoid hemorrhage. The sudden rupturing of a blood vessel may cause loss of consciousness, and the blood may also rupture into the brain, causing neurological disturbances. Often preliminary physical and neurological examinations are completely normal, so the physician who first examines the patient may not consider the condition to be serious. It follows that anyone who has a sudden, severe headache (usually more severe than any pain previously experienced) should go to the emergency room of a hospital and insist on a CAT scan to search for evidence of fresh blood in the head. If the results are negative, a spinal tap may be recommended to check for blood in the cerebrospinal fluid.

When the meninges are irritated by infection, a generalized headache occurs. This condition is known as *meningitis*, and may be either bacterial or viral in origin. Bacterial infections are usually more debilitating and potentially fatal than viral infections. The diagnosis is usually straightforward, in that the patient is commonly very sick and totally disabled, with high fever, severe generalized weakness, nausea, vomiting, and pronounced stiffness of the neck.

Meningitis due to a fungus infection often occurs in people with AIDS. Rarely, cancer may spread to the meninges and cause headache with stiff neck.

Disease of Blood Vessels

Headaches also occur when blood vessels in the head or neck are diseased, a condition that may lead to stroke. Strokes are caused by a rupture of a blood vessel in the brain. This leads to a *brain hemorrhage* or a clot within a blood vessel, which deprives part of the brain of blood, a *brain infarction*. (Hemorrhage within the brain causes headache more often than does a clot blocking an artery.) Generalized or localized symptoms of a stroke depend on the part of the brain that is affected. The headache is usually one-sided and throbbing. Occasionally, it may be a warning of an impending stroke and may occur days or even a week before the event. Since vascular disease of the brain is one of the most common events of aging, underlying organic disease must be considered until proved otherwise when headaches first appear after age 50.

The blood vessels of the head also may become inflamed and cause headaches, a condition that occurs more in arteries than in veins. Inflammation of arteries is referred to as *arteritis;* the inflammation blocks the artery, and the tissue normally supplied with blood by the artery deteriorates. Arteritis may affect only the brain (*cerebral arteritis*), or the brain may be one of many organs affected by generalized or systemic arteritis. When many organs are involved, the most common causes of the arteritis are the

141

collagen diseases; the best known is *lupus erythematosus*. Lupus causes a buildup of collagen (a fibrous protein) that blocks small arteries and thereby injures the organs affected. The diagnosis of lupus must be considered when a stroke affects a young person, with or without disease in other organs.

Temporal arteritis is a low-grade inflammation that originates in the arteries of the scalp, typically the artery that supplies the temple. Also known as *cranial arteritis* or *giant-cell arteritis*, temporal arteritis is a disease of the elderly; it almost never occurs before age 55, and the incidence increases with age. Typically, the patient experiences pain in the temple, but the headache may occur in any part of the head. The pain increases in frequency and often becomes continuous. Initially, there may be no other symptoms, but sometimes jaw pain during chewing is also present. (This has nothing to do with TMJ dysfunction syndrome, which is associated with jaw pain at rest as well as when chewing.) The pain is caused by inflammation of the arteries that supply the muscles of the scalp and the muscles involved in chewing. The inflammation in itself might not be serious, were it not for the fact that other arteries that lie deeper and supply the eyes and brain with blood eventually also become inflamed. If the diagnosis is not made in time, the patient may experience double vision or blindness and may finally develop a stroke.

Often, temporal arteritis is not limited to the head but affects the body as a whole, causing pain and aching that seem to be located in the muscles or joints. This condition is called *polymyalgia rheumatica*. The diagnosis of temporal arteritis is often missed because the results of the standard examination are usually normal. Typically, there is a swollen, reddened, tender artery at the temple where the headache is located, but this is not always the case; or the affected artery may be covered with hair and not readily visible. The patient may or may not have a low-grade fever. When temporal arteritis or polymyalgia rheumatica is suspected, a test is performed that is known as the erythrocyte (red blood cell) sedimentation rate. A high reading supports the diagnosis, which is further confirmed when a simple biopsy of the temporal artery reveals chronic inflammation. (Both tests are performed as outpatient procedures.) The condition responds dramatically to treatment with corticosteroids (prednisone).

Carotidynia is a term applied when pain and tenderness occur on one side of the neck over a carotid artery, one of the main blood vessels in the neck that supplies the brain. This condition usually clears after a week or two. It may be due to a transient inflammation around the carotid artery, but its cause is uncertain.

Rarely, deterioration occurs in the wall of the carotid or vertebral artery, and blood gets into the weakened area and travels along the arterial wall. This *dissection of the carotid or vertebral artery wall* causes pain in the neck, head, or eye. In addition, the artery itself is narrowed or blocked, which often results in a stroke.

Head Injury

Head injury is a common cause of organic headache. Most often, acute pain occurs in the area of the injury, and the pain subsides as the injury heals. In some instances, however, headache persists long after external healing has taken place. In these cases of *post-traumatic headache*, for reasons that are not well understood, the severity of the chronic headache is not correlated with the severity of the injury (see chapter 6).

Whiplash injuries of the head and neck are common, especially when motor vehicles are "rear-ended." Usually no more than neck muscle strain occurs, but when the muscles, ligaments, or tendons of the neck are severely stretched or torn, healing is slow and the associated neck and head pains are prolonged. Whiplash injuries can be even more serious, causing a fractured vertebra or herniated disk. In addition, the shaking of the brain may lead to a post-traumatic headache as part of a post-concussion syndrome.

HEADACHE IN DISEASE AFFECTING THE WHOLE BODY

There are three general causes of headaches that result from diseases of the body as a whole: congestion of blood within the head, a sudden and severe rise of blood pressure, and disorders that affect many organs of the body.

Congestion of Blood in the Head

We noted earlier that an increased volume of material within the confines of the rigid skull casing can cause excessive pressure, resulting in a severe headache. An excess of blood may accumulate in the head when the veins that normally drain the head are obstructed, as in congestive heart failure. Sometimes, too, more blood than normal is pumped into the head—during a convulsion, for example. Blood vessels commonly dilate in response to a fever, to certain toxins (such as carbon monoxide), and to many medications. Often when blood vessels dilate within the head it is in response to an *elevation in the level of carbon dioxide* (CO_2) in the bloodstream, which occurs with lung or heart disease. As in migraine, the dilation itself is not sufficient to cause a headache, but the swelling of the blood vessels probably sets off a series of physiological events that are similar to a migraine attack.

Lack of oxygen at high altitudes often causes headaches and may also cause edema of the lungs or brain. Closer to home, people who tend to sleep with bed coverings pulled up over their heads may decrease oxygen availability and build up a high level of carbon dioxide in their blood. Certain people, especially obese men, have a condition known as *sleep apnea*, when they stop breathing for as long as two minutes during sleep. When apnea occurs, blood oxygenation falls and the level of carbon dioxide in the blood rises. This also occurs with lung disease, with exposure to carbon monoxide, or with any condition that causes insufficient oxygen supply.

Sudden, Severe Hypertension

We have noted that high blood pressure isn't normally a cause of headache, but a very *sudden and severe rise in blood pressure* will initiate a headache. This kind of rapid rise may cause swelling and tiny hemorrhages in the brain, a condition known as *hypertensive encephalopathy*. Sometimes larger hemorrhages occur. The condition is associated with certain tumors of the adrenal gland (*pheochromocytomas*), with the sudden worsening of common high blood pressure, and with a toxic state that sometimes occurs during pregnancy (*eclampsia*).

Certain antidepressants known as MAO inhibitors, for example, phenelzine sulfate (Nardil) or tranylcypromine (Parnate), make patients more susceptible to sudden and severe rises in blood pressure, particularly if they also eat foods such as hard cheeses, herring, sausage, or red wine that contain tyramine. A rapid but brief rise in blood pressure also may accompany sexual intercourse and orgasm. Only rarely, however, does a headache follow (see chapter 4).

Disorders of Many Organs

The third general cause of headache as a result of bodily diseases are *those disorders that affect the head and brain along with many other organs*. These are exemplified by cancers of the lung and breast, which often spread, or *metastasize*, to the brain. In

145

addition, bacteria and toxins can be carried to the brain and all other organs by the bloodstream; generalized infection carried by the blood is called *septicemia* ("blood poisoning"). *Collagen diseases*, such as lupus, also may affect all organs, including the brain.

Metabolic changes often involve the brain and cause headache. Severe hypoglycemia in diabetics who take too much insulin, and biochemical changes in patients undergoing dialysis for kidney failure are particularly associated with headaches. Body toxins that are not properly secreted by the kidneys or properly metabolized by the liver and external poisons, such as contact with large amounts of insecticide, can also affect the brain and other organs.

HEAD, NECK, AND FACE PAIN DUE TO LOCAL DISEASE OR DYSFUNCTION

The preceding sections describe headaches caused by disease in the head and disease in the body as a whole. Here we turn to *localized causes of head and face pain.*

Virtually any disease of the head and/or neck may cause pain. This is especially true in the case of infection, tumor, or injury, and usually these causes of pain are clear. Other conditions affecting the head and neck, however, may not be as obvious, and the diagnosis may be missed. It is these less obvious conditions that we survey here.

Diseases of the Head and Neck

Diseases of the bones of the head and face usually cause pain only when they are infected, as in *osteomyelitis,* or when they are invaded by certain tumors, as in *multiple myeloma.* Many diseases of the neck cause pain in the neck that often extends to the head, especially the back of the head. This is particularly true of *whiplash injuries,* which often occur to the driver or a passenger in a car that is hit from the rear (see page 136). The neck muscles are intimately connected with the scalp muscles, and pain originating in one site can easily extend to the other. When neck muscles are the cause of pain, they are usually found to be tender, and the range of motion of the neck is restricted. (*Arthritis* commonly affects the bones and joints of the neck, but as we have noted, no correlation has been found between the degree of arthritis and the degree of head pain a patient suffers.)

Diseases of the Eye

The diseases of the eye that cause headache are usually obvious. *Acute glaucoma* (excessive pressure within the eyeball), for example, will cause pain in and around the eye, with redness and cloudiness of the cornea. A less severe condition, *subacute glaucoma*, may cause similar pain, but may not show the typical signs. *Nearsightedness, farsightedness,* and *astigmatism* cause us to strain to see better; these refractive errors may cause headache and are correctable with eyeglasses. Sometimes headaches are caused by a *weak eye muscle* or muscles, which result in a squint or "crossed eyes." When suspected, these eye conditions must be confirmed and corrected by an ophthalmologist.

Diseases of the Ear, Nose, and Throat

The most common causes of these diseases are acute infections. *Acute sinusitis* causes fever, nasal congestion, and discharge of pus, in addition to pain and swelling over the affected area, and distinguishes itself sufficiently from other conditions so that the diagnosis should not be difficult (see chapter 6). Chronic sinus infections are much less likely to cause headache. On the other hand, *tumors* within the ear, nose, and throat that may cause head pain usually are not obvious. Although uncommon, they are unfortunately often malignant. Consultation with an ear, nose, and throat specialist is required for correct diagnosis and treatment.

Diseases of the Mouth and Jaw

Of the *diseases of the mouth* that can cause pain of the face and head, an *infected tooth* is the most common. Sometimes an infected molar or impacted wisdom tooth causes a painful sensation that is felt predominantly in the temple rather than in the tooth; this may lead to a mistaken diagnosis of migraine or tension headache (see the case history in chapter 1).

When the *temporomandibular joint* (TMJ) is obviously affected by arthritis, infection, or tumor, or when the joint has been severely injured, pain occurs in and around the TMJ and may extend into the head. Local tenderness may also be present, as well as difficulty in opening the jaw and increased pain when chewing. A dysfunction of the joint is often blamed for the pain, which actually might be caused by spasm in the jaw's muscles (see chapter 6 for a more complete discussion).

DISORDERS AND DISEASES OF THE CRANIAL NERVES OR THEIR BRAIN PATHWAYS

When the cranial nerves or their pathways in the brain are affected, severe pain often results. Disease of the cranial nerves (neuritis) causes a persistent pain, while dysfunction or irritation of these nerves (neuralgia) produces a sharp, momentary stab or series of stabs of pain. The pain caused by disorders of pain pathways in the brain is a continuous burning sensation often described as unlike anything felt before. Physicians term this type of pain *dysesthesia or dysalgesia*.

Neuritis

Headache or eye pain associated with sudden blindness in one eye is usually due to inflammation of the optic nerve, termed *optic neuritis* or *retrobulbar neuritis*. This condition is often associated with multiple sclerosis. Sudden paralysis of an eye muscle results in double vision, a condition that is often caused by *diabetic neuritis* and is associated with local pain. Double vision, with severe pain in the eye, may also be caused by a chronic infection or inflammation (*granuloma*) located behind the eye. This disorder, the Tolosa-Hunt syndrome, responds well to prednisone therapy.

The cranial nerves, as well as nerves in other parts of the body, may be infected by the *herpes zoster* virus, causing the painful condition known as *shingles*. Shingles is most likely to occur in the elderly or in people who have an impaired immune system. The virus often affects the first (ophthalmic) division of the trigeminal nerve of the face, causing a painful blistering around the eye and forehead. Particularly in the elderly, the pain often persists for more than six months. This extended form of the disease is termed *postherpetic neuralgia* and is highly resistant to all forms of therapy. It can, however, usually be partially relieved by a combination of tricyclic antidepressant analgesics (for example, amitriptyline [Elavil]), in combination with a major tranquilizing agent (for example, fluphenazine [Prolixin]).

Neuralgia

The pain of cranial neuralgia is usually excruciating. Cranial neuralgias usually first appear in late middle age or old age. Patients experience sudden, severe, and excruciating knifelike pains in one or more branches of a cranial nerve. The pain lasts only for a moment, but it strikes repetitively, for several seconds, or even for a full minute. On examination, patients with one of the cranial neuralgias demonstrate normal signs; the affected cranial nerve shows no evidence of damage.

The most common form of cranial neuralgia is *trigeminal neuralgia* (also known as tic douloureux because the pain causes the patient to wince, as with a "tic"). While the cranial neuralgias usually appear later in life, trigeminal neuralgia may occur in young people as a symptom of multiple sclerosis. Pain is most common in the branches of the cranial nerves that supply the upper and lower jaw, but also may appear in the area around the eye or forehead. It may be provoked by lightly touching the skin of the face, or by stimulating the mucous membranes of the mouth during eating, drinking, or even yawning. However, sharp pain may also occur spontaneously, without provocation.

Glossopharyngeal neuralgia is a rare condition. Typically, the pain occurs in the throat and extends to the ear; it is provoked by swallowing. *Laryngeal neuralgia* occurs in the throat; *geniculate neuralgia* in the ear.

Sometimes the occipital nerve supplying sensation to the back part of the scalp is pinched by muscles or scar tissue. When this causes pain over the back of one side of the head, it is called *occipital neuralgia*. In contrast to the other cranial neuralgias, the pain is less severe, but it is also more prolonged.

Trigeminal and other cranial neuralgias can be successfully treated with anticonvulsants, the same type of medication that is used for epilepsy. The most commonly used agents are carbamazepine (Tegretol) and phenytoin (Dilantin). If the medication fails to help or, as often happens, if the pain recurs in spite of the medication, neurosurgical procedures are performed to partially damage the nerve and relieve the pain. In patients with trigeminal neuralgia, the surgeon inserts a needle into the face to the root of the nerve and coagulates it with a radiofrequency current or injects glycerol into the area. Alternatively, surgery may be performed to lift away the blood vessel that has caused irritation of the nerve root next to the brain stem. (When the trigeminal nerve is surgically injured in the course of treating trigeminal neuralgia, the affected area of the face may become insensitive to pain, yet the patient may continuously feel a painful burning sensation in this area. This condition is called *anesthesia dolorosa*.) In patients with occipital neuralgia, a simple anesthetic injection (*nerve block*) is often helpful.

Disorders of the Pain Pathways in the Brain

Pain caused by disorders of the pain pathways in the brain is usually continuous, agonizing, and unresponsive to standard pain medication, including morphine and other narcotics. These pains may be ameliorated with a tricyclic antidepressant analgesic in combination with a major psychotropic agent. The mechanisms of these pains are not well understood. Often an injury to a peripheral or cranial nerve initiates the pain, which is then perpetuated in the brain by a complex set of events called *deafferentation*. Anesthesia dolorosa and postherpetic neuralgia, described above, are in this category.

A severely painful or disturbing sensation also may affect the face and other parts of the body when pain centers or pain pathways in the brain are injured by such disorders as stroke or multiple sclerosis. When part of the thalamus, a major relay center for pain that lies deep in the brain, is affected by a stroke, the result is sometimes continuous pain over half of the body or face. This condition is known as the *thalamic syndrome*.

Atypical facial pain, as the name implies, is facial pain that does not conform to any of the conditions noted above. The overwhelming majority of people classified as having atypical facial pain are women, usually in their thirties or forties. The pain is deep in the face, but otherwise not well localized; it is continuous and its quality is often difficult to describe. Since there are no obvious causes for this pain and it is notoriously resistant to all forms of treatment, experts agree that psychological factors are prominent, if not predominant, in this condition.

8

Headaches in Children

Contrary to most beliefs, children are often prone to headaches. The evaluation and treatment of childhood headaches are similar to those we have described in adults, but with certain differences in emphasis. In treating children, it's particularly important for the physician to find out about the young patient's early development, his or her past illnesses, and any family history of similar conditions. The doctor must also inquire into the child's home life and social situation. Are the parents separated or divorced? Does their marriage appear troubled or unstable? Are there hints of physical or psychological abuse? Is the child under any special pressure from family or peers? Does the child have a difficult relationship with teachers? The stresses of developing maturity along with the emerging awareness of sexuality and the struggle for independence that takes place during adolescence may play important contributing roles in the development of headaches. And just as in adults, migraine attacks may be triggered by missing meals, getting too little sleep, or sleeping too much—situations that are common among adolescents.

Very young children may not be able to express their symptoms adequately. It's common for children who can't describe their headache symptoms to be restless and irritable. Because the severity of pain is often difficult for a young child to articulate, it can best be evaluated by the degree to which it interferes with the child's normal activities. If the child is willing to play or to watch television, he or she probably doesn't have a very severe headache. On the other hand, a child with severe migraine will not have to be told to lie down and rest in a quiet, dark room—such a reaction will come spontaneously, as it does to adults. In treating headaches, the same diagnostic tools that are used for adults are applicable to children: a detailed history, a thorough examination, and, if necessary, further tests, such as a CAT scan or MRI of the head.

MIGRAINE IN CHILDREN

Migraine is a common form of headache in children; more than half of adult migraine patients experienced their first attack before the age of 20. In contrast to the particular gender-specific distribution among adults, migraine is reported as frequently among boys under the age of 10 as among girls. The outlook for children with migraine is good: the headaches spontaneously disappear in as many as 50 percent during their teens, and in another 25 percent early in adult life. (Parents who do not themselves experience migraine attacks but have children who do should see chapter 1 for a full description of classic and common migraine.)

The following categories show the wide range of migraine that can affect children; several uncommon variants occur much more frequently in children than in adults. *Ophthalmoplegic migraine*, for example, is a migraine headache accompanied by double vision and is caused by weakness or paralysis of one or more of the muscles involved in eye movement. Double vision may occur during or even after the headache, and may last for days or weeks.

When weakness, paralysis, or numbness of an arm or leg on one side of the body accompanies the headache, the condition is referred to as a *hemiplegic migraine*. Often, the weakness or numbness alternates from one side of the body to the other in subsequent attacks. Approximately half of the children who have these attacks have other family members with a history of a similar condition.

Basilar migraine in children is manifested by symptoms and signs that precede or accompany a migraine headache and affect the base of the brain. Symptoms may include severe unsteadiness of the arms or legs; weakness or numbness of both arms or legs; severe, spinning dizziness; and mood disturbances or loss of consciousness. An *acute confusional state* may occur as part of the attack. The child appears disoriented, restless, or combative, possibly with intermittent drowsiness. Although this condition is often frightening, as with other auras of classical migraine, the symptoms usually disappear within 30 to 60 minutes, but sometimes may last for several hours. The acute confusional state may occur without headache. Similar symptoms are often seen in children who have an infection or have suffered a seizure. The *"Alice in Wonderland" syndrome* is similar to the acute confusional state. The child may complain that everything looks smaller or larger, or is changing in shape; there may be a disturbance in the sense of time, and the child may report odors, sounds, or flavors that are not apparent to others. These symptoms may occur before, during, or after the migraine headache.

Abdominal migraine in children consists of periodic abdominal pain, or nausea and vomiting, or both. Sometimes the abdominal pains are not accompanied by headache, and thus they may constitute a migraine equivalent. The symptoms may last for

155

hours or for days, and the physician must consider and eliminate the diagnosis of abdominal disease before making the diagnosis of abdominal migraine. Another migraine equivalent is *paroxysmal vertigo*, which consists of sudden bouts of severe spinning sensations and a loss of equilibrium. These symptoms occur mainly in children between the ages of two and four; after age four, these children may experience motion sickness and eventually may develop more typical migraine symptoms.

Convulsive seizures may occur more commonly in children with migraine than one would expect on the basis of chance. Headache often follows a convulsion, but differentiating the convulsion from an attack of migraine or other headache is not difficult.

Most migraine headaches that occur in children are the common type, without aura but with nausea and often vomiting. The variants of migraine described above, although more common in children than in adults, are fortunately rare.

TENSION HEADACHES

Occasional tension headaches are common in children, but chronic daily headaches also occur. The symptoms are similar to those experienced by adults (see chapter 2). In most instances, the headaches are traceable to psychological stress that is related to problems with family, school, or peers. The headaches may be a sign of depression or other mood changes, or evidence of anxiety. While the depression may not be obvious, it is often manifested by deterioration in schoolwork; difficulty in falling asleep or, conversely, excessive sleeping; aggression and irritability; withdrawal from social contact; weight loss or, less commonly, weight gain. Children with chronic tension headaches typically miss many days of school and, subconsciously, may be using the headaches to gain sympathy and attention or to avoid responsibilities.

CLUSTER HEADACHES

The very painful condition known as cluster headaches is fortunately quite rare in children. If and when these headaches do occur, they have the same characteristics as those encountered by adults (see chapter 3).

TREATMENT

The successful treatment of headaches in children is usually less difficult than in adults. Often they require no more than psychological reassurance, the removal of triggering factors, and the judicious use of over-the-counter pain relievers. Sometimes, a sedative or antinauseant may be recommended. Note: *Aspirin can be dangerous in young children, as it has been associated with Reye's syndrome, a potentially fatal illness that affects the liver and brain; Reye's syndrome may itself begin with a headache.* Because of this, aspirin for children is avoided, and acetaminophen (for example, Tylenol) is usually used as an analgesic. In contrast to adult treatment, prescribing pain medications for children during the early stages of a headache may be unwise, since the medication may mask other symptoms that might assist in making the diagnosis.

Because of the relative infrequency of their attacks, most children with migraine don't require preventive medication, so this kind of daily medicating can usually be avoided. If preventive medication is necessary, all the medications recommended for adult migraine patients may be used (see chapter 1), with the important exception of methysergide maleate—its potential side effects are too dangerous to risk in children. Because it has few side effects, cyproheptadine (Periactin) is often used to prevent childhood migraine. The anticonvulsants, such as phenytoin, are sometimes beneficial; slurred speech, unsteadiness, and drowsiness are their most common potential adverse side effects. As with adults, all these medications should be used only under a doctor's supervision. Remember that children learn relaxation and biofeedback techniques more quickly and easily than adults, so these therapies may be used in place of or as a supplement to medication.

HEADACHE DUE TO UNDERLYING DISORDERS

Naturally, the parents of children who suffer from headaches are particularly concerned about the possible presence of serious underlying disease, especially a brain tumor. If your child has recurring or occasional particularly severe headaches, remain calm. The chances are overwhelmingly against the cause being a brain tumor. Despite the benign statistical perspective, though, any severe headache that does not disappear requires medical attention. Although organic diseases account for a very small percentage of headaches in children, they must always be the physician's first consideration.

Of the organic disorders that can produce headache in children, the most important are the many diseases of childhood that can cause increased pressure in the head. This pressure may be the result of a *brain tumor* or *abscess*, a *subdural hematoma* (a clot between the brain and the skull), a blockage with enlargement of the ventricles of the brain (*hydrocephalus* or "water on the brain"), *meningitis*, *encephalitis*, and *swelling of the brain*.

Symptoms of the above conditions can be unsteadiness, weakness, sleepiness, deterioration in schoolwork, personality changes, and convulsive seizures. (An unexplained deterioration in schoolwork is often the first evidence of cognitive change in a child.) Unexplained vomiting, especially without preceding nausea, may be caused by excessive pressure in the head. Any of these symptoms, as well as any local neurological signs affecting strength, sensation, or vision that accompany headache, warrant immediate medical attention.

A headache alone may be a clue to the presence of underlying disease. Headaches of recent origin are more worrisome than those that have recurred for many years; occasional headaches that take place over a long period of time are more likely to be migraine or tension headaches. Another sign of a serious disorder may be headaches that awaken a child in the middle of the night or headaches that are aggravated by straining or head movements, or a head pain that is consistently located in one particular area of the head (this, of course, can also be a symptom of migraine). A change in the pattern of chronic headaches is also an indication of possible underlying disease.

Increased pressure in the head is not always due to such serious diseases as brain tumors. A condition known as *pseudotumor cerebri* ("false tumor of the brain") is sometimes seen in adolescents who are overweight, young women who have menstrual problems, or both. This disorder is due to swelling of the brain, which causes the excessive intracranial pressure. It is characterized by headaches that become continuous and at first are unaccompanied by any other symptoms. An eye examination, however, will reveal the swelling of the ends of the optic nerve (papilledema). Pseudotumor cerebri is usually benign and will eventually clear, but it must be treated to prevent damage to the optic nerve, which can lead to loss of vision.

Certain other much more common disorders of the head and neck can cause headaches in children. The *common cold*, with an upper respiratory tract infection, is often associated with headache, as are *infections of the ear*, particularly the middle ear (behind the ear drum). *Tooth decay and abscess* may cause frontal or temporal headaches in children as well. The sinuses around the nose are not well developed in very young children, but as they grow older *acute sinusitis* can occur, with pain over the front of the head and between the eyes accompanied by nasal congestion and drainage. A history of hay fever or other allergies may also be present. Children are particularly susceptible to *fever*, which can cause headaches. In addition, almost any *toxic reaction*, such as inhaling or consuming external poison or an internal biochemical change, will provoke headaches in children.

The Parents' Role

As is obvious from the previous list of potentially serious conditions sometimes found in children, you as a parent should always pay attention to your child's headache symptoms. Try to find out where the pain is located, when it started, what it feels like, and whether your child has ever experienced a similar type of headache before. If the headache lingers, or if headaches recur frequently or with sufficient severity to disrupt the child's daily activities, see a physician promptly.

In the case of chronic headaches, you need to pay special attention to the role of stress in your child's life. Are you making unrealistic demands on your child? Are there serious problems at home, at school, with playmates? Not all stress can be eliminated, of course, but certain difficult situations can be rectified or modified with or without professional help. Your physician can advise you on how to control your child's headaches and whether further therapy is needed.

9

Headaches in
the Elderly

It has been estimated that more than 10 percent of all elderly people experience headaches of one type or another. Most headaches in the elderly are benign, and are due either to migraine, tension headache, or cluster headache. Although these headaches may begin at any age, the vast majority start in adolescence and in young adult life; however, they may persist into middle age and beyond.

Migraine headaches, for one, typically decrease in frequency and severity after midlife. Most women with migraine find that their headaches subside after menopause. However, there are some who experience a worsening of migraine attacks with menopause and, rarely, migraine may begin at that time. As people with classical migraine (migraine with aura) grow older, they may find that the aura symptoms continue to recur, but often without the subsequent headache. These are considered *migraine equivalents*. In some instances, migraine equivalents can begin in mid- and late adult life. In these cases, when a headache does not follow the

161

symptoms of the brain disturbance that make up the aura, the symptoms are likely to be confused with transient cerebrovascular disease. The difference lies with the onset of the symptoms. The aura of migraine gradually evolves in its intensity and extent over a period of 20 or 30 minutes, whereas a *cerebral transient ischemic attack (TIA)* is usually sudden in onset or reaches its maximum intensity within a few minutes.

Tension headaches, like migraine, tend to subside in midlife and especially in the elderly, but sometimes persist into old age and rarely begin at that time. Chronic tension headaches, especially chronic daily headaches, are prone to persist for decades, since these headaches sometimes become a way of life. While *cluster headaches* usually begin between the ages of 20 and 40, they are more likely to begin in the fourth, fifth, or sixth decade of life than are migraine or tension headaches. The characteristics of migraine, tension headaches, and cluster headaches tend to be the same in the elderly as in young people.

Psychological factors are no more likely to cause headache in the elderly than in younger people. On the other hand, depression associated with the many psychological traumas to which one is increasingly exposed during life may evoke headaches. These factors include chronic illness either in the patient or the spouse, or the death of the spouse or a close relative. Other emotional problems associated with the family or work have been found to be prominent in older patients who have benign headaches. For example, displacement from the comforts of one's home is, unfortunately, not rare. Abuse of alcohol or drugs is less often associated with headaches in the elderly than in young adults.

Although most headaches beginning in late life are due to a change in the function rather than in the structure of tissues in the head, the doctor's primary concern is the possibility of underlying structural organic disease (see chapter 7).

HEADACHE DUE TO UNDERLYING DISEASE

Of the diseases within the head, a *brain tumor* is the first consideration. Indeed, the prevalence of brain tumors markedly increases in the sixth and seventh decades of life. Similarly, *cerebral aneurysms* tend to increase in size and vulnerability of rupture as one grows older. Thus, *subarachnoid hemorrhage* is more common in mid- and later life than in youth. *Cancer* is also more common in the elderly and metastasis to the brain or the meninges, most often from the breast or lung, may signal its presence by headaches.

Vascular disease due to *hardening of the arteries (atherosclerosis)* is another manifestation of the aging process and can lead to a stroke, either due to blockage or breakage of a blood vessel within the brain. A headache may precede the stroke by days or a week and accompanies cerebral hemorrhage more often than cerebral infarction. *Temporal arteritis* virtually never begins before the age of 55. It is a major consideration when headache begins in the elderly and it is readily responsive to therapy. Prednisone, administered early in the course of the temporal arteritis, can prevent the complications of blindness and stroke.

As one grows older, the brain tends to shrink and one becomes more vulnerable to the development of a *blood clot (subdural hematoma)* between the brain and the skull. Whenever the head is moved, there is slight movement of the brain within the confines of the skull. Such movement puts some degree of stress on the veins that drain blood from the brain and pass through the skull. With increasing space between the skull and the brain, there is the increasing danger of a shearing effect on these bridging veins. Thus, an insignificant bump of the head may cause the rupture of one or more of these veins and the development of a blood clot in the area. This subdural hematoma tends to gradually increase in size until it compresses the brain. Headache with increasing drowsiness and impairment of mental function are more common features of this condition than focal signs of brain disturbance.

Because illness often accompanies aging, diseases that affect the body often cause headache in the elderly. *Heart failure* and *lung disease* may result in vascular congestion in the head and so may lead to headache. *Sleep apnea* is common in middle-aged men, particularly those who are obese; morning headache with daytime drowsiness are symptoms of this condition. While the prevalence of high blood pressure increases with age, common forms of hypertension are not associated with headache (popular belief to the contrary notwithstanding). But people taking a monoamineoxidase inhibitor medication for depression may experience a sudden and severe rise in blood pressure if they disobey their doctor's advice and eat foods containing tyramine, such as hard cheese, or take medication that interacts with the antidepressant. A sudden and severe rise in blood pressure from any cause is usually associated with headache and may lead to cerebral hemorrhage.

All of the local diseases that cause pain in the head or face (see chapter 7) must be considered when headaches begin in the elderly. *Arthritis* is another one of those diseases that almost inevitably occur as part of the aging process. As noted, however, the degree of arthritis affecting the neck does not correlate with the occurrence or degree of pain of the neck and head. *Glaucoma* is the most common eye disease of the elderly and, in the acute phase, causes pain in and around the eye. Older people are subject to *periodontal disease* rather than tooth cavities; the pain of associated infection is usually localized to the affected part. Infections and tumors affecting the ears, nose, and sinuses are not significantly more common in the elderly than in the younger population. However, the bone tumor (*multiple myeloma*) usually occurs after the age of 40 or 50; it is a rare cause of headache.

For reasons not well understood, several disorders of the cranial nerves are more common in the elderly than in the younger population. The incidence of *shingles* (*herpes zoster*) rises with age; approximately half of the people who live to 85 years of age have experienced one attack. More than 10 percent of all cases are *ophthalmic herpes*, that is, they involve the ophthalmic division of the trigeminal nerve carrying pain sensation from the area of the eye and the forehead. *Postherpetic neuralgia*, the persistence of pain for more than 6 months, occurs in half of the patients after the age of 60 and the incidence continues to rise with increasing age.

Except for those people who have multiple sclerosis, *trigeminal neuralgia* and the other cranial neuralgias usually begin later in life. Many researchers believe that trigeminal neuralgia is caused by a blood vessel (adjacent to the nerve root) that has become tortuous with age. The repeated pulsations of the artery eventually injure the nerve and set off the complex pain mechanism. The *thalamic syndrome* is a rare cause of head and face pain in the elderly. It is usually due to a stroke that has affected portions of the thalamic nucleus of nerve cells deep within the brain.

Grim as some of these illnesses are, it must be emphasized that most headaches in the elderly are *not* due to serious disease. Migraine, tension headaches, and cluster headaches that persist into late life are amenable to treatment. Similarly, those headaches due to organic disease disappear or diminish with the correction of the underlying condition.

10

Should You See a Doctor?

Obviously, there's no need to consult a physician every time you have a headache—95 percent of headaches are *not* due to serious disorders. Many of the more serious symptoms associated with headaches and described in this chapter, for example, also occur during attacks of migraine, particularly nausea, vomiting, and visual disturbances. What follows is intended to provide you with a context for exercising your own good judgment about when to seek medical advice.

HEADACHES WARRANTING
A DOCTOR'S ATTENTION

If you experience headaches that appear to be a component of the specific diseases described in chapter 7 of this book, then medical attention is strongly recommended. Particularly, if you experience a sudden and severe headache, more severe than anything you've encountered in the past, see a physician or go to an emergency room immediately.

Sudden onset of very severe head pain is typical of a ruptured cerebral aneurysm. With such a rupture, blood pours into the subarachnoid space, the area between the brain and the skull. The blood may not injure the brain directly, but the increased pressure within the skull causes a severe headache. Loss of consciousness may accompany the initial rupturing of the aneurysm. If blood ruptures into the brain, weakness, numbness, or visual impairment on one side occurs. Not every severe headache or sudden onset of head pain is due to a ruptured aneurysm, but the danger of missing the diagnosis is so great that immediate medical attention is necessary. A CAT scan of the head, a spinal tap, or both may be needed to establish or rule out this diagnosis.

When a headache becomes progressively worse over a period of weeks or months, it is time to see a doctor. Such a headache may increase in severity, frequency, and duration until it becomes continuous. The progressive worsening of any neurological condition may be a sign of an expanding mass within the head, such as a brain tumor, abscess, or blood clot. Usually these conditions will cause distinct neurological symptoms, such as weakness, disturbances in sensation, or abnormalities in vision. These neurological signs may be so subtle, however, that you may not recognize them; they may become apparent only during a physician's examination.

A third type of headache that warrants consulting a physician is *the persistence of headache after head or neck injury.* Headache is common after such injuries, but it usually disappears after a few hours or a day or so. Even when the headache persists for more than a week, it is not necessarily due to severe injury or disease. A whiplash injury of the neck, for example, may strain ligaments and muscles, causing prolonged neck and head pain. On the other hand, prolonged headache after an injury may be due to the formation of a blood clot between the brain and skull, a subdural hematoma. This type of blood clot tends to increase in size gradually, causing the buildup of pressure within the head and localized pressure on the brain. Sometimes the blood clot grows large enough to shift the brain within the skull, causing coma and death. Just before this happens, the pupil of one eye dilates and becomes unreactive to light. However, no one should wait for these signs to emerge before seeking medical attention. Extreme severity of a headache or duration of head pain for more than one week is sufficient reason to see a doctor.

A fourth type of headache that requires medical attention is a *recurrent or persistent headache that first appears in late middle age or later in life.* As we have seen, most benign headaches such as migraine or tension headaches begin in adolescence or young adult life. When headaches begin later in life, they are often a component of underlying disease rather than functional disturbance of blood vessels or muscles. One uncommon but readily treated disorder that begins after age 55 is temporal or cranial arteritis (see chapter 7). This inflammatory disease first affects blood vessels of the scalp, and later extends to the blood vessels that supply the eye and the brain. If this condition is recognized promptly, treatment with corticosteroids can produce almost immediate resolution.

There are two further situations in which the symptoms that accompany headache warrant a physician's attention. These pertain to *symptoms referable to the nervous system* and *symptoms that affect other parts of the body.* Nervous system symptoms accompanying headaches may be either localized, generalized, or both. Weakness or numbness of an arm or leg on one side, difficulty in seeing in one direction, or a tendency to fall in one direction are common examples of localized neurological symptoms and usually indicate that disease of the brain is underlying the headache. Generalized neurological symptoms that may accompany headache and indicate disease within the head include drowsiness, failing memory, and changes in personality or behavior. A convulsive seizure may precede, accompany, or follow localized or generalized neurological symptoms. The symptoms may indicate a brain tumor or other mass, the impending or early stage of a stroke, or a toxic or inflammatory process in the head—encephalitis or meningitis for example.

Of the large number of symptoms referable to the body, relatively few, when associated with headache, warrant a physician's attention. *Fever* with headache may be due to no more than a common cold. But if there is no simple explanation—in particular, if the headache becomes increasingly severe—you should consult a physician. The combination of headache and fever may be caused by such serious illnesses as encephalitis, meningitis, or endocarditis, as well as by more common, minor illnesses. *Shortness of breath* associated with headache may be caused by lung disease or heart failure. *Vomiting* with headache is a dangerous sign if it is sudden and *not* preceded by nausea; such spontaneous vomiting may be an indication of increased pressure within the head. Nausea with vomiting, on the other hand, is commonly due to an upset stomach. *Excessive fatigue* when associated with headache may indicate the presence of serious disease, such as cancer or arteritis. But again, this common symptom usually occurs in relation to benign and much less threatening conditions.

When symptoms referable to the eyes accompany a headache, an ophthalmologist should be consulted, just as symptoms referable to the ears, nose, and throat warrant the attention of an otolaryngologist (ear, nose, and throat specialist). While relatively minor diseases of these structures may be associated with headache, so may serious conditions such as glaucoma or acute sinus infection that warrant prompt medical attention. Common sense dictates that symptoms referable to the mouth and teeth require a dentist's attention, whether or not they are associated with headache.

In principle, you should also consult a physician if your headaches do not respond to over-the-counter analgesics. You may, in fact, be taking an excessive amount of these medications and causing a rebound headache. Or perhaps you have undiagnosed migraine or cluster headaches that warrant prescription medication.

Keep in mind, too, that any change in the customary pattern of headaches you may have experienced in the past may indicate the presence of a new underlying disease. This is sufficient reason to consult a physician. As a general rule, if your headaches are interfering with your relationships with family or friends or with your ability to work or study, or if the pain is simply preventing you from enjoying life, see a doctor.

THE PHYSICIAN'S ROLE

In all fields of medicine, successful treatment depends on establishing the correct diagnosis. For the physician, the most important aspect in establishing the diagnosis of your headache is a detailed history of your symptoms. Your doctor will need to know all the facts about your headaches:

- At what age—or on what occasion—did the headaches start?
- At what time of day or night do they occur?
- How long do the headaches last?
- How often do they occur?
- Where is the headache located when the pain begins, and where does it extend to as it develops?
- What is the nature of the pain—throbbing, a steady ache, sharp?

- How severe is the pain—mild, moderate, or severe, or as graded on a scale from 1 to 10?
- What, if any, symptoms occur before, during, and after the headache? Do you have visual; ear, nose, and throat; or gastrointestinal symptoms? Do you have symptoms that are referable to your scalp, face, jaw, or neck? Are your symptoms referable to the brain or your involuntary nervous system, such as sweating or cold hands? Be specific.
- What particular factors appear to trigger or aggravate your headaches? If you are female, is there any relationship between menstruation or pregnancy and the occurrence of your headaches? Are the headaches aggravated by physical activity or emotional stress? Do changes in the weather affect them? What foods, drinks, or medications aggravate or trigger your headaches?
- What measures give you partial or complete relief? For example, do you prefer to lie still in a dark, quiet room, or to move about during a headache?
- What has been the course of your headaches? Are they getting better, worse, or are they fluctuating without basic change?
- What medications have you taken in the past, and what, if any, are you currently taking? (This query refers to both prescription and nonprescription drugs.) Include all the medications that have *not* worked in the past, along with their dosages. (This information may prevent the re-prescribing of previously ineffective medication, or indicate the necessity for a higher dosage than in the past.)

It is always helpful to bring a record of all past medical tests, so that these are not needlessly repeated.

In addition to the history of the headache itself, your physician will want to know as much as possible about your present and past state of health—past illnesses, surgery, and injuries—as well as to review other symptoms that might be referable to the nervous system and the rest of the body. You'll also be asked about the medical history of other people in your family, particularly close relatives.

Finally, your doctor will inquire about your daily habits: whether you smoke or drink and how much. Information about your family, work, and outside interests may also be important. He or she will try to get some impression of your personality and moods. Do you seem anxious or depressed, for example? Many patients who don't realize that they're depressed may report alterations in their sleeping patterns, appetite, or sexual drive, or show other symptoms that are indications of depression.

After taking this detailed history, the doctor will examine you. In addition to obtaining your vital signs, such as pulse and blood pressure, and giving you a standard physical examination, a neurological exam will be conducted. This exam consists of an evaluation of your mental faculties, the external condition of your neck and head, examination of your cranial nerves (which control eye movement and facial expression and sensation), examination of your motor system and basic coordination, evaluation of sensation, and tests of your reflexes. In the great majority of headache patients, the results of all these tests will be normal.

It's important to note that the physical and neurological examinations, as well as any laboratory tests, are *not* performed to establish a diagnosis of migraine, tension headache, or cluster headache. No tests can establish these diagnoses. Rather, their purpose is to determine whether an underlying disease is the cause of your headaches, since some disorders may mimic the symptoms of migraine, tension headache, or cluster headaches.

In the past, patients with headaches also underwent routine X rays of the skull, electroencephalography, and imaging tests, such as isotope brain scan. It was found that the routine use of these tests was not cost-effective—the results were usually normal and serious diseases, such as a brain tumor, were found very rarely. Besides, serious disorders are usually revealed by the medical history and the examination; when necessary, the diagnosis is corroborated by relatively new and far more elaborate tests. Among them are two that show details of the brain with marvelous clarity: *computerized tomography* (known as CAT or CT scan) and *magnetic resonance imaging* (MRI). Noninvasive and usually quite safe, these procedures are, nevertheless, expensive to perform, costing hundreds of dollars.

Ideally, every headache patient seen by a doctor should undergo one of these tests, but they rarely reveal disease that would not have been evident by other means. In practice, if a patient has a history typical of migraine, tension headache, or cluster headache, and the physical and neurological examinations are normal, it's neither necessary nor practical to put him or her through the expense of a CAT scan or MRI of the head. If an unusual factor turns up in the medical history or examination, one of these tests is warranted.

Other tests do sometimes show interesting changes in patients with migraine, tension headaches, and cluster headaches. These tests include *electroencephalography* (EEG), *thermography* (which depicts different temperature zones on the face), and *transcranial Doppler studies* (which measure changes in velocity of blood in major head arteries, denoting narrowing of the arteries as in spasm). None of these tests are of value in diagnosing benign headaches, however, and they, too, are usually unnecessary. Their primary value rests in research.

Occasionally, additional tests *are* necessary. Sometimes the patient requires a *spinal tap* to look for blood or inflammation as the cause of a severe sudden headache. Rarely, the patient may require hospitalization to have *arteriography* (known also as *angiography*) performed. This test outlines the blood vessels of the neck, head, and brain after a contrast material is injected into the arteries at the base of the neck. (A similar procedure is used in heart patients to examine the coronary arteries.) Arteriography can detect an aneurysm or other vascular disorders as well as spasm or inflammation of the arteries that are not usually found by other means.

A Family Practitioner or a Specialist?

For experienced practitioners, the diagnosis and treatment of most headaches is not particularly difficult. If your family physician spends the time to take a detailed history and establish the correct diagnosis, he or she should be able to help you. However, if your headaches persist, the attention of a neurologist or internist is appropriate.

If the condition still persists after treatment by these specialists, you may decide to go to a headache clinic that offers a multidisciplinary approach to treatment. The primary specialist—usually a neurologist—works with other professionals who are highly experienced in treating and counseling headache patients. In addition, the clinic usually includes on its staff the services of a psychologist or psychiatrist and a biofeedback technologist. Dentists, ophthalmologists, and ear, nose, and throat specialists are usually available to the headache-clinic patient for consultation, and the clinic's personnel meet periodically to discuss difficult cases and present the latest research. Even though patients who visit headache clinics often come with particularly difficult diagnostic and therapeutic problems, the professionals at this type of clinic can usually help considerably.

Why would they be able to help you, especially if other treatments have failed? Physicians who specialize in one field develop a body of experience and knowledge of their subject and can focus on those details in diagnosis and treatment that may make the difference between failure and success. Accustomed to seeing every variation in headache patterns, they are trained to consider every aspect of the patient—the social and psychological along with the medical—and so achieve a high rate of success with their patients.

When Hospitalization Is Necessary

At times, it is necessary to hospitalize patients even if it's been established that they are suffering from migraine, cluster headaches, or tension headaches rather than headaches caused by a serious underlying disease. Hospitalization may be required when an attack of migraine is unusually severe, incapacitating, and prolonged, as in status migrainosus (see chapter 1). Once in the hospital, the patient receives intravenous fluids to replace fluid and mineral loss from vomiting. He or she may also receive intravenous or intramuscular injections of DHE 45 (ergotamine tartrate), meperidine (Demerol), prochlorperazine (Compazine), or metochlopramide (Reglan) to break the prolonged migraine attack.

On extremely rare occasions, the aura (the localized neurological signs) of migraine is prolonged. If these signs last more than a week, the patient is considered to have suffered a migrainous stroke. Because the stroke may have occurred coincidentally, hospitalization is necessary both to look for causes of the stroke other than migraine and to treat the stroke itself.

Some people with chronic cluster headaches fail to respond to any of the presently available medications. Hospitalization may be recommended to treat these patients with a course of intravenous histamine or, as a last resort, to destroy (by means of radiofrequency coagulation) the first branch of the trigeminal nerve, which carries the pain message (see chapter 3).

As we have seen, people with chronic tension headaches often take excessive amounts of over-the-counter or prescription medications that may perpetuate their headaches on a rebound basis. Most people can be helped to gradually discontinue these daily medications as outpatients. Sometimes, however, patients have become habituated or addicted to these medications and cannot withdraw from them on their own. In such cases, they must be hospitalized and undergo a period of detoxification.

A few headache clinics offer hospital beds that are devoted exclusively to patients with headaches. In addition to the specific treatments noted here, patients in these hospital headache units may be seen by a physical therapist, a dietician, a biofeedback technician, and a psychologist or psychiatrist in order to start them on a course of nonpharmacological therapy in addition to whatever medication is warranted.

Setting Goals

It's important for you and your physician to *set certain goals* with regard to what you expect from successful treatment, and to be specific about what that entails. Rarely can headaches be "cured" in the sense of your never suffering through one again. But even though the underlying tendency for recurrence remains, most headaches can be prevented for long periods, and those that do occur can be substantially diminished in intensity. Indeed, the object of any therapy selected by you and your physician should be to decrease the frequency and severity of your headaches to a degree that will allow you a normal life-style.

If you've read this book, you know that there is no reason for you to continue to suffer with headaches. If the headaches are interfering with your life in any way, it's time to seek relief by consulting with a physician. Hopefully, the headaches that were once a major disruption will become an occasional minor nuisance. That certainly is success by any measure.

REFERENCES

INTRODUCTION

Friedman, A. P. "Headache in History." *Bulletin of the New York Academy of Medicine* 48 (1972): 661–81.

Headache Classification Committee of the International Headache Society. "Classification and Diagnostic Criteria for Headache Disorders, Cranial Neuralgias and Facial Pain." *Cephalalgia* 8 (Suppl 7) (1988): 1–96.

Linet, M. S., W. F. Stewart, D. D. Celentano, D. Ziegler, and M. Sprecker. "An Epidemiologic Study of Headache Among Adolescents and Young Adults." *Journal of the American Medical Association* 261 (1989): 2211–16.

Sigerist, H. E. *A History of Medicine*. Vol. 1, *Primitive and Archaic Medicine*. New York: Oxford University Press, 1955.

Waters, W. E. *Headache*. Littleton, Mass.: PSG Publishing, 1986.

1. MIGRAINE HEADACHES

Blau, J. N. "Adult Migraine: The Patient Observed." In *Migraine: Clinical and Research Aspects*, edited by J. N. Blau. Baltimore: Johns Hopkins University Press, 1987, 3–30.

Diamond, S., ed. *Migraine Headache Prevention and Management.* New York: Marcel Dekker, 1990.

Gowers, W. R. *A Manual of Diseases of the Nervous System.* London: J & A Churchill, 1892.

Sacks, O. *Migraine: Understanding a Common Disorder.* Los Angeles: University of California Press, 1985.

Sandler, M., and G. M. Collins, eds. *Migraine: A Spectrum of Ideas.* New York: Oxford University Press, 1990.

Selby, G. *Migraine and Its Variants.* Boston: ADIS Health Science Press, 1983.

Solomon, S., K. Guglielmo-Cappa, and C. R. Smith. "Common Migraine: Criteria for Diagnosis." *Headache* 28 (1988): 124–29.

2. TENSION HEADACHES

Bakal, D. A., and J. A. Kaganov. "Muscle Contraction and Migraine Headache, Psychophysiologic Comparison." *Headache* 17 (1977): 208–15.

Langemark, M., and J. Olesen. "Pericranial Tenderness in Tension Headache." *Cephalalgia* 7 (1987): 249–55.

Langemark, M., J. Olesen, D. L. Poulsen, and P. Beck. "Clinical Characterization of Patients with Chronic Tension Headache." *Headache* 28 (1988): 590–96.

Mathew, N. T., E. Stubits, and M. Nigam. "Transformation of Migraine into Daily Headache: Analysis of Factors." *Headache* 22 (1982): 66–68.

Pritchard, D. W. "EMG Cranial Muscle Levels in Headache Sufferers Before and During Headache." *Headache* 29 (1989): 130–38.

Takeshima, T., and K. Takahashi. "The Relationship Between Muscle Contraction Headache and Migraine: A Multivariate Analysis Study." *Headache* 28 (1988): 272–77.

3. CLUSTER HEADACHES

Ekbom, K. "A Clinical Comparison of Cluster Headache and Migraine." *Acta Neurologica Scandinavica* 46 (Suppl 41) (1970): 7–48.

Kudrow, L. *Cluster Headache: Mechanisms and Management.* New York: Oxford University Press, 1980.

Mathew, N. T., ed. *Cluster Headache.* New York: SP Medical & Scientific Books, 1984.

Sjaastad, O., and I. Dale. "A New (?) Clinical Headache Entity 'Chronic Paroxysmal Hemicrania.'" *Acta Neurologica Scandinavica* 54 (1976): 140–59.

Solomon, S. "Cluster Headache and the Nervus Intermedius." *Headache* 26 (1986): 3–8.

4. HEADACHE TRIGGERS

Blau, J. N., F. R. C. Path, and M. Thavapalan. "Preventing Migraine: A Study of Precipitating Factors." *Headache* 28 (1988): 481–83.

Dalton, K. "Food Intake Prior to a Migraine Attack—Study of 2,313 Spontaneous Attacks." *Headache* 15 (1975): 188–93.

Van den Bergh, V., W. K. Amery, and J. Waelkens. "Trigger Factors in Migraine: A Study Conducted by the Belgium Migraine Society." *Headache* 27 (1987): 191–96.

5. NONDRUG THERAPIES

Adler, C. S., S. M. Adler, and R. C. Packard. *Psychiatric Aspects of Headache.* Baltimore: Williams & Wilkins, 1987.

Bakal, D. A., S. Demjen, and J. A. Kaganov. "Cognitive Behavioral Treatment of Chronic Headache." *Headache* 21 (1981): 81–86.

Benson, H. *Beyond the Relaxation Response*. New York: Berkeley, 1984.

Brown, J. M. "Imagery Coping Strategies in the Treatment of Migraine." *Pain* 18 (1984): 157–67.

Schwartz, M. S., et al. *Biofeedback: A Practitioner Guide*. New York: Guilford Press, 1987.

Sorbi, M. *Psychological Intervention in Migraine*. Delft, The Netherlands: Eburon, 1988.

6. CONTROVERSIAL HEADACHES

Ayer, W. A. "Report of the President's Conference on the Examination, Diagnosis and Management of Temporomandibular Disorders." *Journal of the American Dental Association* 106 (1983): 75–77.

Bennion, L. J. *Hypoglycemia: Fact or Fad*. Mount Vernon, N.Y.: Consumers Union, 1983.

Edmeads, J. "The Cervical Spine and Headache." *Neurology* 38 (1988): 1874–78.

Kottke, T. E., J. Tuomilehto, P. Puska, and J. T. Solonen. "The Relationship of Symptoms and Blood Pressure in a Population Sample." *International Journal of Epidemiology* (1979): 355–59.

Levin, H. S., H. M. Eisenberg, and A. L. Benton, eds. *Mild Head Injury*. New York: Oxford University Press, 1989.

Friedman, W. H., and B. N. Rosenbaum. "Paranasal Sinus Etiology of Headache and Facial Pain (Review)." *Otolaryngologic Clinics of North America* 22 (1989): 1217–28.

7. HEADACHES DUE TO DISEASE

See general references.

Headache Classification Committee of the International Headache Society. "Classification and Diagnostic Criteria for Headache Disorders, Cranial Neuralgias and Facial Pain." *Cephalalgia* 8 (Suppl 7) (1988): 1–96.

Solomon, S., and R. B. Lipton. "Facial Pain." In *Neurologic Clinics: Headache*, edited by N. T. Mathew. Philadelphia: W. B. Saunders, 1990.

Solomon, S., and R. B. Lipton. "Atypical Facial Pain: A Review." *Seminars in Neurology* 8 (1988): 332–38.

8. HEADACHES IN CHILDREN

Barlow, C. F. *Headache and Migraine in Childhood*. Philadelphia: J. B. Lippincott, Oxford Blackwell Scientific Publications, 1984.

Labbe, E. E. "Childhood Muscle Contraction Headache." *Headache* 28 (1988): 430–34.

Prensky, A. L. "Migraine in Children." In *Migraine: Clinical and Research Aspects*, edited by J. N. Blau. Baltimore: Johns Hopkins University Press, 1987, 31–53.

Shinnar, S., and B. J. D'Souza. "The Diagnosis and Management of Headaches in Childhood." *Pediatric Clinics of North America* 29 (1982): 79–94.

9. HEADACHES IN THE ELDERLY

Cook, N. R., D. A. Evans, H. H. Funkenstein, P. A. Scherr, A. M. Ostfeld, J. O. Taylor, and C. H. Hennekens. "Correlates of Headache in a Population-Based Cohort of Elderly." *Archives of Neurology* 46 (1989): 1338–44.

Fromm, G. H., C. F. Terrence, and J. C. Maroon. "Trigeminal Neuralgia: Current Concepts Regarding Etiology and Pathogenesis." *Archives of Neurology* 41 (1984): 1204–07.

Loeser, J. D. "Herpes Zoster and Post Herpetic Neuralgia." *Pain* 25 (1986): 149–64.

Portenoy, R. K., C. J. Abissi, R. B. Lipton, A. R. Berger,

M. F. Mehler, J. Boglivo, and S. Solomon. "Headache and Cerebrovascular Disease." *Stroke* 15 (1984): 1009–12.

Poser, C. M. "The Types of Headache that Affect the Elderly." *Geriatrics* 31 (1976) (Sept): 103–106.

Solomon, S., and K. Guglielmo-Cappa. "The Headache of Temporal Arteritis." *Journal of the American Geriatric Society* 35 (1987): 163–65.

10. SHOULD YOU SEE A DOCTOR?

See general references.

GENERAL REFERENCES

Dalessio, D. J. *Wolff's Headache and Other Head Pain.* 5th ed. New York: Oxford University Press, 1987.

Diamond, S., and D. J. Dalessio. *The Practicing Physician's Approach to Headache.* 4th ed. Baltimore: Williams & Wilkins, 1988.

Headache Classification Committee of the International Headache Society. "Classification and Diagnostic Criteria for Headache Disorders, Cranial Neuralgias and Facial Pain." *Cephalalgia* 8 (Suppl 7) (1988): 1–96.

Lance, J. W. *Mechanism and Management of Headache.* 4th ed. Boston: Butterworth Scientific, 1982.

Raskin, N. H. *Headache.* 2nd ed. New York: Churchill Livingstone, 1988.

Saper, J. R. *Headache Disorders: Current Concepts and Treatment Strategies.* Boston: John Wright PSG, 1983.

INDEX